THE MEDICAL MARIJUANA DISPENSARY

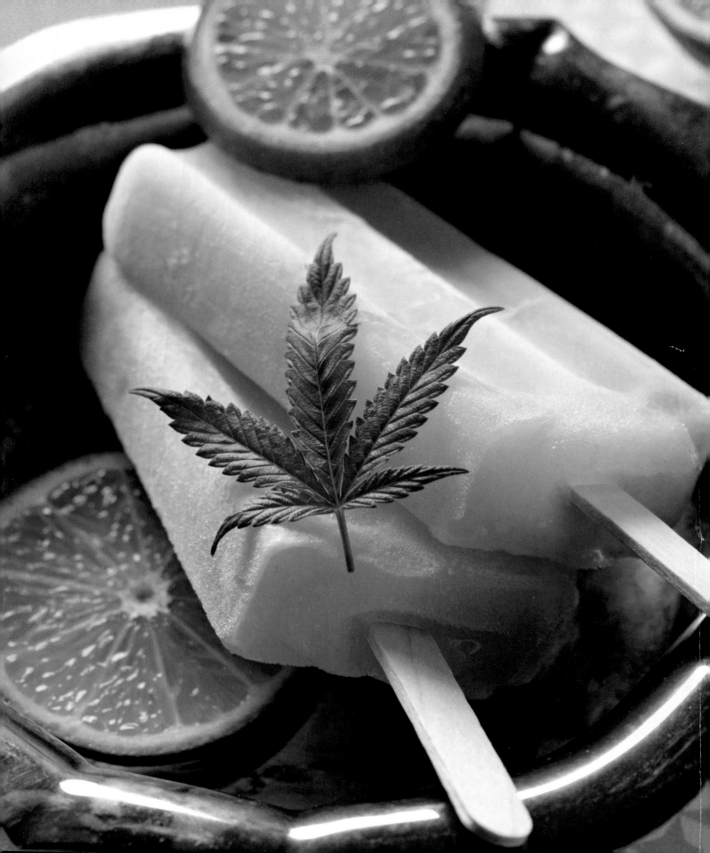

THE MEDICAL MARIJUANA
DISPENSARY

Understanding,
Medicating, and Cooking
with Cannabis

LAURIE WOLF and MARY WOLF

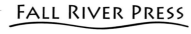

FALL RIVER PRESS

New York

FALL RIVER PRESS

New York

An Imprint of Sterling Publishing Co., Inc.
1166 Avenue of the Americas
New York, NY 10036

ISBN 978-1-4351-6811-4

For information about custom editions, special sales, and premium and corporate purchases,
please contact Sterling Special Sales at 800-805-5489 or specialsales@sterlingpublishing.com.

Manufactured in China

2 4 6 8 10 9 7 5 3

sterlingpublishing.com

CONTENTS

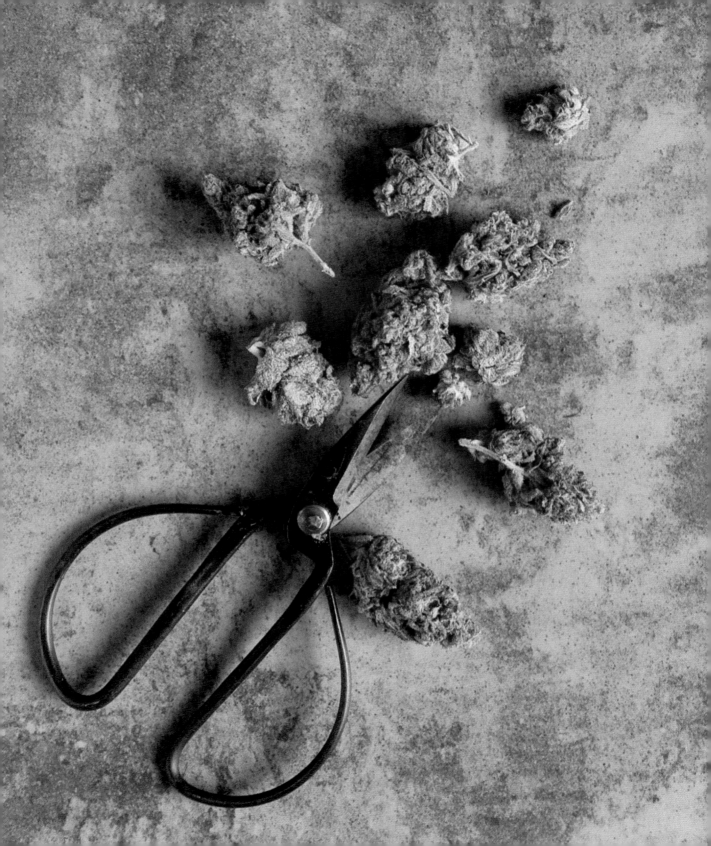

FOREWORD

PAUL ARMENTANO

Deputy Director of NORML

IF YOU ARE reading this book, there's a good chance you are new to cannabis. However, cannabis is not new to you. Humans have cultivated and consumed the flowering tops of the female cannabis plant, colloquially known as marijuana, since virtually the beginning of recorded history. Cannabis-based textiles dating back to 7000 BCE have been recovered in northern China, and the plant's use as a medicinal, spiritual, nutritional, and mood-enhancing agent dates back nearly as far.

Modern cultures continue to utilize the cannabis plant for these same purposes, despite its stigmatization and criminal prohibition over the better part of the past century. In the United States, Congress first outlawed cannabis in 1937 by passing the Marihuana Tax Act of 1937. Federal lawmakers doubled down on cannabis prohibition in 1970 by classifying the plant, and all of its biologically active organic compounds, as Schedule I controlled substances. This flat-Earth position alleges that cannabis's risks to health are equal to those of heroin, and that the plant possesses "no currently accepted medical use in the United States,"[1] according to the official definition of a Schedule I drug.

The National Organization for the Reform of Marijuana Laws (NORML) initially challenged this classification in 1972. As a result of this legal suit, in 1988 the US Drug Enforcement Administration's own administrative law judge opined, "Marijuana, in its natural form, is one of the safest therapeutically active substances known to man"[2] and ordered the plant to be rescheduled. The agency ultimately rejected this order and, in the years since, has disallowed a series of additional legal challenges, stating that cannabis fails to possess therapeutic efficacy and has not been accepted as a treatment option by qualified experts.

---

1. United States Drug Enforcement Agency, "Drug Scheduling," accessed December 27, 2015, www.dea.gov/druginfo/ds.shtml.
2. Francis L. Young, "In the Matter of Marijuana Rescheduling Petition; Docket No. 86-22" (September 6, 1988), accessed January 2, 2016, www.ccguide.org/young88.php.

This stance is woefully out of step with public, medical, and scientific opinion. Recent polls indicate that upward of 85 percent of Americans believe that cannabis ought to be legal when authorized by a physician,[3] while nearly 60 percent of voters endorse permitting the plant's use to anyone over the age of 21.[4] Twenty-three states and Washington, DC, have enacted legislation authorizing cannabis therapy. Four states have elected to regulate the plant's commercial production and sale to all adults. And another 15 states have taken steps to permit the use of cannabidiol, a distinct plant cannabinoid known for its anticonvulsant activity, by qualified patients.

Health professionals are also becoming increasingly comfortable with the use of cannabis as a viable treatment option, particularly as an alternative to opioid painkillers. In fact, data published in the *Journal of the American Medical Association* finds that opiate-related mortality is significantly lower in states where medical cannabis is permitted as compared to states where the plant remains prohibited.[5] Medical associations like the American Nurses Association and the Epilepsy Foundation of America are on record in support of providing patients with safe, legal access to cannabis. A 2014 WebMD survey reported that nearly 7 in 10 physicians,

including over 80 percent of oncologists, believe that cannabis provides legitimate therapeutic benefit to their patients.[6]

Science substantiates their opinions. Unlike conventional pharmaceuticals, the cannabis plant enjoys a long history of human use, thus providing society with ample empirical evidence as to its relative safety and efficacy. Moreover, despite cannabis's modern-day politicization, the plant and its compounds have nonetheless been subject to extensive scientific scrutiny. A search using the term *marijuana* on PubMed.gov, the website of the United States National Library of Medicine, yields more than 22,000 scientific papers referencing the plant or its constituents. By comparison, a keyword search using the term *hydrocodone* (a commonly prescribed opioid) yields fewer than 1,000 citations, and a search using the term *Adderall* (a frequently prescribed stimulant for ADHD patients) yields fewer than 200 total papers.

Among this extensive body of literature are over 100 controlled clinical studies evaluating the safety and efficacy of cannabis and its components in various patient populations. A 2012 review of recent FDA-approved trials of herbal cannabis, published in the scientific publication *The Open Neurology Journal*, concludes, "Based on evidence currently

3. "Fox News Poll: 85 Percent of Voters Favor Medical Marijuana," *Fox News*, May 1, 2013, www.foxnews.com/politics/interactive/2013/05/01/fox-news-poll-85-percent-voters-favor-medical-marijuana/. **4.** Jeffrey M. Jones, "In U.S., 58% Back Legal Marijuana Use," *Gallup*, October 21, 2015, www.gallup.com/poll/186260/back-legal-marijuana.aspx. **5.** Marcus A. Bachhuber, "Medical Cannabis Laws and Opioid Analgesic Overdose Mortality in the United States, 1999–2010," *JAMA Internal Medicine* 174, no. 10 (October 2014): 1668–73, media.jamanetwork.com/news-item/lower-opioid-overdose-death-rates-associated-with-state-medical-marijuana-laws/. **6.** R. Scott Rappold, "Legalize Medical Marijuana, Doctors Say in Survey," WebMD, April 2, 2014, www.webmd.com/news/breaking-news/marijuana-on-main-street/20140225/webmd-marijuana-survey-web.

available the Schedule I classification [for cannabis] is not tenable; it is not accurate that cannabis has no medical value, or that information on safety is lacking."[7]

As you read this book, it will become apparent that the US government hasn't been upfront with you about the cannabis plant. Cannabis does not deserve its Schedule I restrictive status; it is not lacking in safety or therapeutic utility. It is also untrue that the science surrounding cannabis, its mechanisms of action and humans' relationship with it, is not well understood. In reality, we as a society know plenty about cannabis, as well as about the failures of cannabis prohibition. It's time to allow people the option to consume a botanical product that is objectively safer than the litany of pharmaceutical and recreational substances it could replace.

Paul Armentano *is the deputy director of the National Organization for the Reform of Marijuana Laws (NORML), and also serves on the faculty of Oaksterdam University in Oakland, CA. He is the coauthor of* Marijuana Is Safer: So Why Are We Driving People to Drink? *(Chelsea Green Publishing, 2013) and the author of* The Citizen's Guide to State-By-State Marijuana Laws *(Whitman Publishing, 2015).*

---

7. Igor Grant, "Medical Marijuana: Clearing Away the Smoke," *Open Neurology Journal* 6 (May 2012): 18–25, www.ncbi.nlm.nih.gov /pmc/articles/PMC3358713/.

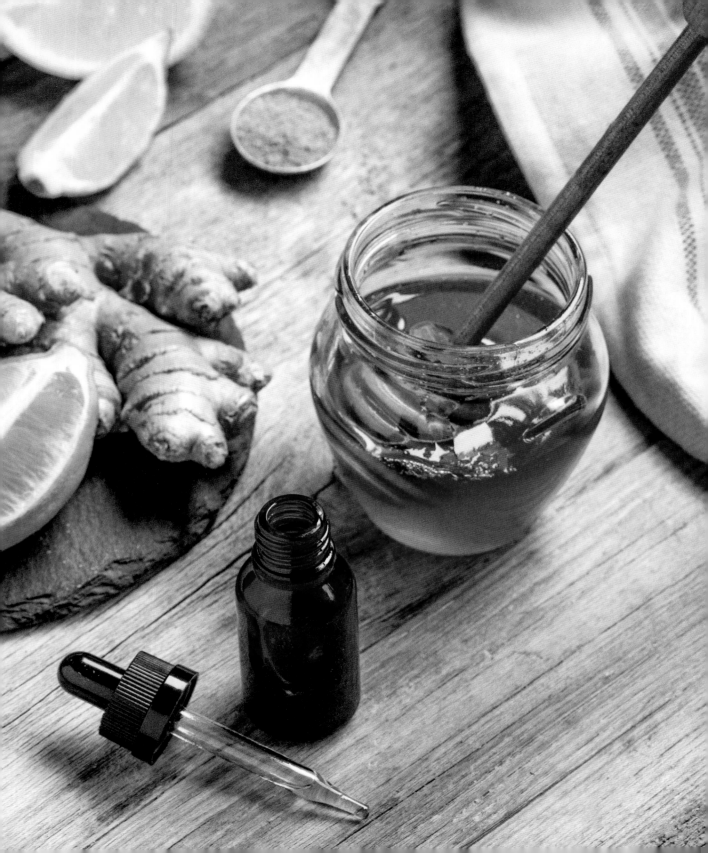

INTRODUCTION

LAURIE WOLF

WELCOME TO THE fascinating and ever-growing world of medical cannabis! I'm glad you're here. Chances are you've heard about the benefits of marijuana for a particular ailment and it has piqued your curiosity. That's how it started with me and many other medical users.

After 20 years, I have finally been able to successfully treat my seizure disorder with marijuana. Before I started using marijuana to treat my condition, I was on several extremely unpleasant prescription medications with horrible side effects, and I still continued to have epileptic auras. At a dinner party, I was introduced to a man with the same condition who was able to manage the disease by using medical marijuana. Within three weeks of medicating with cannabis, I was both aura- and seizure-free. This has been a huge improvement in my quality of life. The frequency at which I have heard stories like mine is astounding. People all over the world are finding relief through cannabis.

There is a growing amount of information and attention around the use of marijuana as medicine. Some of it is perfectly valid; some of it is untested. For anyone new to the field and interested in the therapeutic effects of cannabis, finding accurate, useful information can be a bit daunting. Mary and I put this book together as a way to accumulate and share information and evidence from experienced medical professionals and researchers, as well as contributions from the medical marijuana community. We want this to be a user-friendly manual and guide for anyone who is interested in exploring the world of medical marijuana, so sit back and enjoy the journey!

If you live in a state that allows you to have cannabis, you'll be able to choose your own strain, grow your own marijuana or buy it from a dispensary, and use it in the form you prefer . . . lucky you! If you're not in one of these states, have you considered moving? I'm joking, of course. What you can do is contact the National Organization for the Reform of Marijuana Laws (NORML) to find a local chapter and see what actions you can take to help make marijuana a legal medical option in your state.

As a producer of edibles for the medical community, I have seen compelling results that have led me to believe in marijuana as a medicine, without hesitation. That said, I'm not suggesting that people turn to cannabis for all their medical issues. Many people get relief using cannabis, but there are many conditions that require traditional medical treatment. I'm also not advocating that anyone stop taking their medication and switch to cannabis. Always speak with your doctor before making any changes to your healthcare treatment. It certainly helps to be informed, and that's where this book comes in.

As you make your way through these pages, I hope you find the answers you're looking for. I also hope you come up with questions to ask your doctor and the workers (or budtenders) at any dispensary you visit. Mary and I will discuss the medical issues that are currently being treated with medical marijuana, and we'll shed some light on the specific cannabis strains and their beneficial effects. You will also learn how to figure out the right dose for you and your preferred delivery method. Also included are guides on infusing cooking oils and preparing food with cannabis. The recipes and remedies are simple, effective, and nutritious.

I strongly believe that helping people improve their quality of life and treat their ailments with cannabis is the most important aspect of this "green rush." Helping folks feel comfortable using medical marijuana is my goal.

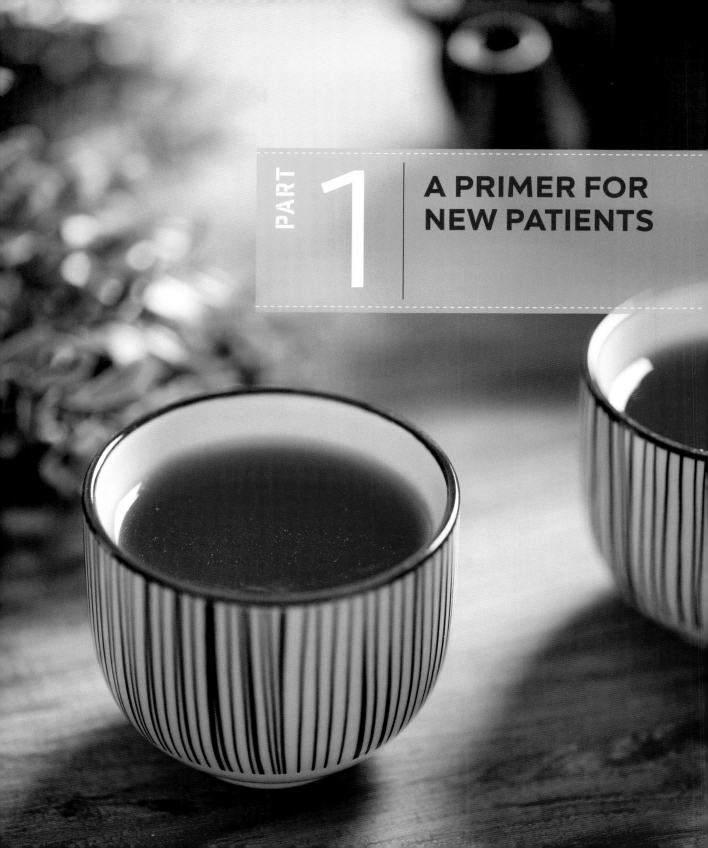

PART 1 | A PRIMER FOR NEW PATIENTS

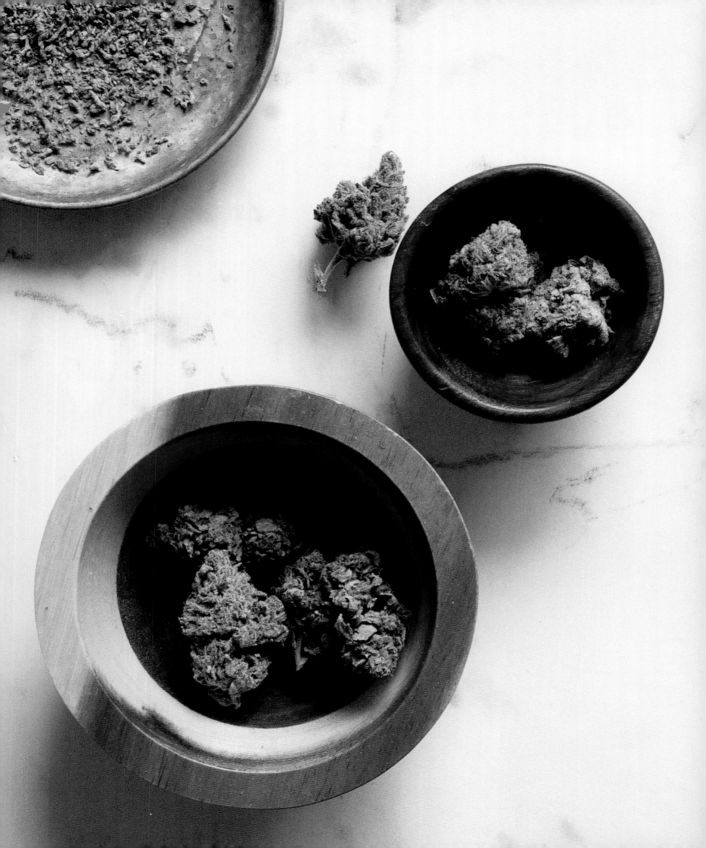

CHAPTER ONE

MEDICAL MARIJUANA DEMYSTIFIED

CANNABIS EXISTED ON this earth long before we did. One of the oldest cultivated crops, it has proven to be a resilient and extremely versatile plant. Not only can it be used to create useful material goods, but it can also aid in the treatment of cancer, Alzheimer's disease, posttraumatic stress disorder (PTSD), multiple sclerosis (MS), amyotrophic lateral sclerosis (ALS), nausea, HIV and AIDS, Crohn's disease, glaucoma, epilepsy, and a growing list of other health conditions. While new research continues to emerge on an almost daily basis, there is still a long way to go to fully understand the many benefits of this amazing plant.

CANNABIS BASICS

" *I am very glad to hear that the Gardener has saved so much of . . . the India Hemp . . . The Hemp may be sown anywhere.*"
—**George Washington**, first president of the United States, in a letter to his farm manager, William Pearce, in February 1794

The amazingly useful cannabis plant has been growing on this planet long before humans learned of its benefits. Outside of its medical and recreational usage, cannabis is used to make textiles, rope, fiber, paper, biofuel, and food. In fact, the word *canvas* comes from the root word *cannabis*. As its common nickname *weed* might indicate, this plant can be grown just about anywhere as long as it is exposed to a consistent temperature that is not too cold and has adequate light and food.

Cannabis is a flowering plant that includes at least three species: *sativa*, *indica*, and *ruderalis*. (*Sativa* and *indica* are the species profiled in this book; *ruderalis* is not commonly grown in the United States for medicinal purposes.) The plant is an annual, meaning it completes its life cycle within one year. It is also dioecious, meaning that male and female organs are found on separate plants, although some plants can become hermaphroditic under certain conditions. The female plant produces the flower, or the *buds,* as they are known in the cannabis world. The flowers are the richest source of the chemical compounds in cannabis, so the males, which produce the pollen, are generally used just for breeding purposes.

The Parts of the Plant

Marijuana plants can be male, female, or both. Females produce the flowering buds, while males produce pollen. When pollinated, the female will produce seeds. This also reduces the quantity of buds. Males are isolated or destroyed unless breeding or seed production is the goal. Fan leaves extend off the stem up until the main cola, or terminal bud. The bud, or calyx, has the highest concentration of trichomes. Trichomes are resin-filled glands that contain THC.

People primarily use the bud for medicinal purposes. You can also use shake, or small pieces of bud. The iconic fan leaves are the least potent and generally aren't used. Small leaves close to the buds, called sugar leaves, are useful in extractions. Just like buds, they are coated in trichomes. The stem isn't very potent, but it does contain cannabidiol (CBD). The stem is used in commercial hemp production.

On average, a marijuana plant takes 3 to 4 months to mature for harvesting. After harvest, the flowers are prepared for their intended use, whether it be via smoking, vaping, ingesting, or topical application. If the plant is going to be smoked, the bud will be dried and cured before it is ready. If you're going to use a vaporizer, you will use ground-up, dried buds or an oil concentrate (extraction) made from the cannabis buds. Many people prefer vaporizers because there is no harsh smoke; the vapor is generally cool and easy on the lungs. If you intend to use the cannabis for cooking, the buds are generally cooked in butter or oil. As they cook, tetrahydrocannabinol (THC) and other cannabinoids are released and attach to the fat in the oil or butter. Cannabinoids are the active chemical compounds in marijuana. Tinctures can be made for oral ingestion by steeping the cannabis in alcohol or vegetable glycerin. For easy recipes and remedies you can make at home, go to part 3 of this book.

Cannabis goes by many names; the most common are marijuana, hemp, and hash. Names for cannabis are always changing. Throughout its history, it has been known by a wide range of interesting slang terms such as weed, grass, dope, bud, pot, maryjane, skunk, schwag, kush, wacky tobaccy, bhang, dank, herb, reefer, chronic, weird, sticky-icky, cheeba, ganja, and Aunt Mary (a personal favorite of ours). As you'll soon discover, the various strains have some interesting names as well.

Popular Uses of Cannabis

When most people think of marijuana, they think of its recreational use. But ancient records also point to industrial, medicinal, and ceremonial uses of marijuana by many cultures throughout history. The same range of applications for cannabis continues today.

Industrial   Hemp, a nonpsychoactive variety of cannabis, is made from the stalk of the plant. It's a renewable resource used in thousands of products. Considered the world's oldest domesticated crop, it can be used to make paper, rope, fabric, biofuel, beauty products, and food. Cannabis came to the New World on the *Mayflower*—hemp fiber had been used to make the ship's sails and ropes, and hemp seeds were in the cargo. The colonies were actually required to grow hemp because of its necessity to everyday life. In fact, the Declaration of Independence and Betsy Ross's American flag were both made of hemp. In 1970, the Controlled Substances Act banned all forms of cannabis, even hemp, by classifying it as a Schedule I controlled substance. However, the Agricultural Act of 2014 made it possible for states to regulate their own hemp legislation. States such as Kentucky, Colorado, and Oregon are already growing this renewable, sustainable, and versatile product.

Ceremonial

The use of cannabis in a ceremonial and spiritual context dates back many thousands of years. In India, a drink of cannabis, milk, nuts, and spices was consumed at the Hindu festival Holi to celebrate the god Shiva, who, as legend goes, created cannabis from his own body. Taoist texts from the fourth century mention using cannabis in incense vessels for meditation and spiritual needs.[8] Ancient German pagans associated cannabis with Freya, the goddess of love. It was believed that Freya lived in the flowers of the plant, and by ingesting them, one possessed Freya's divine powers.[9] In modern culture, the Rastafari movement has embraced cannabis as a sacrament and consider it to be the tree of life. Anecdotally, many people today use cannabis for meditative purposes.

Recreational

Marijuana is the third most popular recreational drug in the world, just behind alcohol and tobacco. In the United Sates, the percentage of people who report smoking marijuana has doubled over the last decade. While many of these people are using cannabis for medical purposes, most are recreational users. That means they use cannabis for its psychological and physical effects, which include relaxation, euphoria, introspection, and creativity. Four states—Washington, Oregon, Colorado, and Alaska—along with the District of Columbia have legalized the recreational use of marijuana. A 2015 poll revealed that 58 percent of Americans believe marijuana should be legal, the third year in a row that the majority has been in favor of legalization.[10]

Medical

One of the oldest written records of cannabis use dates back to 2700 BCE in China, in the form of an ancient healing book. The ancient text indicates the use of cannabis in treating a number of disorders, including rheumatism, gynecological disorders, and absentmindedness.[11] In the late 1800s, cannabis became available at drugstores across the United States in liquid and hashish form. In fact, an 1862 edition of

---

8. Joseph Needham, *Science and Civilisation in China: Volume 5, Chemistry and Chemical Technology, Part 2, Spagyrical Discovery and Invention: Magisteries of Gold and Immortality* (Cambridge University Press, 1974), 150. **9.** Jeffrey Winterborne, *Medical Marijuana Cannabis Cultivation: Tree of Life at the University of London* (Pukka Press, 2008), 289. **10.** Jeffrey M. Jones, "In U.S., 58% Back Legal Marijuana Use," *Gallup*, October 21, 2015, www.gallup.com/poll/186260/back-legal-marijuana.aspx. **11.** David T. Brown, *Cannabis: The Genius Plant* (Amsterdam, The Netherlands: Harwood Academic Publishers, 2003), 1.

For the last six months my dog has been eating dog biscuits made with marijuana. We give her one in the morning and another in the late afternoon. They cost about 50 cents a biscuit. The vet suggested we try her on marijuana because she is allergic to the pain-relieving pills made for dogs. When we rescued her, we knew she had bad hips and was already starting to have trouble walking. But her condition got bad fast, and we were so upset to discover that the traditional medication made her sick. The biscuits have been working very well; in fact, the difference is huge. I might try to make the biscuits myself after doing some research. I have never tried marijuana, and I can hardly believe that my dog is the one in the family uses it. —**Richard S.**, Oregon

Vanity Fair advertised a hashish candy for the treatment of nervousness, weakness, confusion, and melancholy. "Under its influence all classes seem to gather new inspiration and energy," it boasted.[12] When we talk about marijuana in this book, our focus is on its use to treat or prevent a wide range of health issues, from reducing nausea and stimulating appetite to relieving pain and easing muscle spasms . . . and much more.

In 2015, there are 23 states plus the District of Columbia with medical marijuana programs. A person must apply for a medical marijuana card with records of an approved illness from a physician recommending cannabis as a treatment. See the Medical States section (page 23) for a list of states with medical marijuana programs. Doctors can't legally "prescribe" cannabis, as it is still classified as a Schedule I drug, but they can recommend its use.

Profiling Cannabis

When you enter a dispensary, you'll generally notice three main categories of cannabis: *sativa, indica,* and hybrid. Hybrids can be further categorized into *sativa*-dominant hybrids, *indica*-dominant hybrids, or split hybrids. Until very recently, it was believed that *sativas* have energizing, uplifting effects, *indicas* impart more relaxing, full-body therapeutic experiences, and hybrids create observable effects that fall between the two.

But when it comes to the efficacy of medical marijuana, there is an emerging school of thought that believes the classifications of *sativa, indica,* and hybrid are not as important as we have come to believe over the past several decades. In fact, some contend that the differences we experience between *sativas* and *indicas* are a result of the placebo effect and confirmation bias. "The data shows that *indica* and *sativa* is just morphology," said Jeffrey Raber, PhD, in an interview with *LA Weekly.* "It's a misperception that *indica* will put you to sleep or that *sativa* is more energetic."[13] In an analysis of 494 flower samples, Dr. Raber found no evidence that strains

---

12. *Vanity Fair,* Volume 5, January 4, 1862. **13.** Dennis Romero, "Marijuana Strains Like OG Kush Are Meaningless, Experts Say," *LA Weekly,* December 3, 2013, www.laweekly.com/news/marijuana-strains-like-og-kush-are-meaningless-expert-says-4173909.

labeled *indica* and strains labeled *sativa* were chemically distinct entities.[14]

Nevertheless, in today's marijuana market, cannabis plants are still largely classified as *indicas*, *sativas*, or hybrids, and as new consumers, you'll need to be familiar with the way cannabis strains are presented. Because of this, we follow conventional *indica, sativa,* and hybrid classifications when we walk you through profiles of various strains in part 2 of this book.

It is also important to be aware that some growers and sellers may accidentally or even purposely mislabel a strain with a more popular strain name to increase sales and revenue. (Yes, some strains are more expensive than others.) Additionally, the same strain between two growers may have widely differing observable effects, due to variations in climate, soil, light, and food. When picking out a strain to try, remember that you cannot accurately base your selection solely on the *indica, sativa,* hybrid classification or the individual strain's name. Instead, it may be more helpful to focus on other ways of identifying the strain's benefits, such as the breakdown of chemical compounds found in the strain.

The emerging thought today is that the range of effects produced from different cannabis strains comes down to the levels of cannabinoids and terpenes, the chemical compounds found in the plant's resin secreted by the trichomes. "There are biochemically

The Naming of a Strain

Once just referred to as "bud," the list of commercially available strains today is huge and increases with each new harvest. Every strain originates as a unique plant that is crossbred over many generations. Some names describe the genetics and effects of the plant, while others are feats in pure creativity. Don't be put off by some of the strange names. It isn't the name of the strain that matters, but the beneficial effects the strain can impart. There is really no way to verify that a strain you are purchasing actually originated from the source plant, but reputable dispensaries will make an effort to ensure the authenticity of their products and label them appropriately.

distinct strains of Cannabis, but the *sativa/indica* distinction as commonly applied in lay literature is total nonsense and an exercise in futility," reported Ethan Russo, MD, a world-renowned cannabis researcher, in a recent interview with the journal *Cannabis and Cannabinoid Research*. "It is essential that future commerce allows complete and accurate cannabinoid and terpenoid profiles to be available," advises Dr. Russo.[15]

The best-known cannabinoid in cannabis is tetrahydrocannabinol (THC), the compound responsible for the plant's

---

14. S. Elzinga, J. Fischedick, R. Podkolinski, and J. C. Raber, "Cannabinoids and Terpenes as Chemotaxonomic Markers in Cannabis," *Natural Products Chemistry & Research* 3 (2015): 181. doi:10.4172/2329-6836.1000181. **15.** D. Piomelli and E. B. Russo, "The *Cannabis sativa* versus *Cannabis indica* Debate: An Interview with Ethan Russo, MD," *Cannabis and Cannabinoid Research* 1: no. 1 (January 2016), 44–46, doi:10.1089/can.2015.29003.ebr.

psychoactive effects. However, it's merely one of an estimated hundred compounds that we know of. Quickly gaining popularity is cannabidiol (CBD), a nonpsychoactive compound that possesses anticonvulsant, anti-inflammatory, and antianxiety properties and actually counteracts the high from THC. Current medical research is focusing on CBD in the treatment of epilepsy, Crohn's disease, PTSD, and multiple sclerosis. Cannabigerol (CBG) is also growing in importance. CBG has been shown to kill cancer cells and inhibit tumor growth, and may help treat glaucoma and inflammatory bowel disease.[16]

Although recent research has focused on the cannabinoids of marijuana, terpenes are the next frontier. Like cannabinoids, terpenes are oily compounds secreted from the trichomes of the plant. They give different cannabis strains their distinct smells. Unlike the marijuana-specific cannabinoids, terpenes can be found throughout the natural world in our fruits, vegetables, herbs, and spices. We already consume them every day (black pepper, anyone?). There are more than 200 different terpenes found in cannabis, and the terpene profile of a particular strain is thought to play a role in that strain's effects. For example, myrcene is a terpene found in many strains and is known to be a sedative, muscle relaxer, and painkiller. It is also used for its anti-inflammatory effects. In addition to marijuana, it can be found in sweet basil, thyme, lemongrass, hops, and mangos. One cannabis strain that is high in myrcene is White Widow.

Despite the new focus on cannabinoids and terpenes, many people still have strong preferences for certain *sativas* or *indicas*. You might think of it like a preference for red wine over white wine. It can be as simple as that!

THE STATE OF MEDICAL MARIJUANA TODAY

" *[Marijuana] doesn't have a high potential for abuse, and there are very legitimate medical applications. In fact, sometimes marijuana is the only thing that works . . . It is irresponsible not to provide the best care we can as a medical community, care that could involve marijuana. We have been terribly and systematically misled for nearly 70 years in the United States, and I apologize for my own role in that.*" —**Dr. Sanjay Gupta**, neurosurgeon and CNN chief medical correspondent[17]

Humans have been cultivating and medicating with cannabis for thousands of years. As mentioned earlier, records from 2700 BCE show the documentation of more than 100 medical uses for cannabis.[18] Today, we continue to use cannabis for some of these

16. F. Borrelli et al., "Beneficial Effect of the Non-Psychotropic Plant Cannabinoid Cannabigerol on Experimental Inflammatory Bowel Disease," *Biochemical Pharmacology* 85, no. 9 (May 2013): 1306–16, doi:10.1016/j.bcp.2013.01.017. **17.** Sanjay Gupta, "Why I Changed My Mind on Weed," *CNN*, August 8, 2013, www.cnn.com/2013/08/08/health/gupta-changed-mind-marijuana/. **18.** Alison Mack and Janet Joy, *Marijuana as Medicine? The Science Beyond the Controversy* (Washington DC, National Academy Press, 2001): 14–15.

same conditions, despite a federal ban. Cannabis prohibition in the United States began with the Marihuana Tax Act of 1937 and was later reaffirmed with the Schedule I classification in 1970. The most restrictive of the five categories, Schedule I puts cannabis on the same level as heroin, ecstasy, and LSD and classifies it as being more dangerous than cocaine, opium, and meth, all Schedule II substances. This doesn't make any sense.

By definition, Schedule I drugs are substances with a high potential for abuse and no recognized medical or health benefit. Ever since cannabis received this designation, advocates have been working hard to "reschedule" it to a lower tier. Recent efforts to reclassify cannabis have fallen short, despite its legalization by four states and the nation's capital. Although federal law prohibits the use and sale of marijuana, the Obama administration has not made criminal prosecution in legal or partially legal states a "top priority."[19]

Today, the majority of Americans are in favor of legalizing marijuana. Where there is a majority, federal reform can't be far behind. The legalization, or at the very least, the reclassification of cannabis, comes with a number of benefits. The ability to regulate cannabis allows for quality control, potency regulation, proper labeling, and pesticide-testing requirements. In states that have legalized the recreational use of marijuana,

A Word of Caution
Current federal law prohibits you from buying or using marijuana, even if your state has legalized it. Be sure to follow all of the guidelines set forth by your state and use medical marijuana responsibly. For more information, check with NORML at norml.org/legal.

we've seen a drastic improvement in the quality of cannabis. Patients and the public know the type and strength of what they are getting because the information is right there on the label. On the other hand, in states with no medical marijuana program, there is absolutely no control. Patients who choose to pursue cannabis on their own must depend on their supplier for quality assurance and honesty. By legalizing cannabis, an illicit enterprise becomes the territory of doctors, chemists, patients, and business owners—from the black market to the stock market, if you will.

Because the legal landscape for marijuana in the United States is changing rapidly, it is best to visit norml.org/laws for the most up-to-date information on marijuana laws in your state. The information that follows is current as of January 2016.

19. Devin Dwyer, "Marijuana Not High Obama Priority," *ABC News*, December 14, 2012, abcnews.go.com/Politics/OTUS/president-obama-marijuana-users-high-priority-drug-war/story?id=17946783.

Safe and Responsible Use

Before you purchase medical marijuana, be aware of all applicable state laws on what is and is not permitted. States have differing possession limits, home cultivation restrictions, and marijuana concentrate allowances. Responsible cannabis use is important to avoid legal troubles, as well as for the legalization effort. When others witness responsible use, their views might shift. Follow these six principles of responsible cannabis use.

1. ADULTS ONLY

Marijuana is for adults, ages 21 and up. It's irresponsible to give it to children unless otherwise recommended by a qualified doctor for state-approved conditions and after obtaining a medical marijuana card.

2. NO DRIVING

Don't drive while impaired by cannabis, just as you wouldn't drive under the influence of alcohol or prescription medications that cause psychomotor impairment (which is when thinking is slowed and physical movements are reduced). Be smart.

3. PERSONAL LIMITS

Be aware of your personal limits and environment. Don't put yourself or others in any danger or unpleasant conditions.

4. RESIST ABUSE

The use of cannabis to the extent that it impairs health or personal development is considered abuse. Know your limits and stop before exceeding them.

5. RESPECT RIGHTS OF OTHERS

When medicating with marijuana, be aware and respectful of your environment and those around you. Don't violate the rights of others. Those around you may wish to avoid cannabis, including its smoke, entirely.

6. AVOID ADDICTION

Some research suggests that cannabis users may have the potential to develop dependence on marijuana over time. THC releases dopamine in the brain, which can trigger an addiction circuit. Regular cannabis use has also been shown to cause withdrawal symptoms in 40 percent of users when they quit.[20] Working with professionals to get advice on dosage and frequency of usage can be valuable in reducing your risk for addiction and withdrawal.

---

20. David A. Gorelick et al., "Diagnostic Criteria for Cannabis Withdrawal Syndrome," *Drug and Alcohol Dependence* 123, no. 1–3 (June 2012): 141–47, doi:10.1016/j.drugalcdep.2011.11.007.

If you don't live in a state with a medical marijuana program and choose to pursue cannabis as a medical treatment, you must be very cautious. Restriction to patients in need is the worst outcome of marijuana prohibition; while we don't endorse illegal activity, we know that there are those of you who want to use this plant for medicinal purposes. Above all, stay safe. If you're buying from a source without a license to sell, be sure to choose one that is smart, cautious, and has your best interests in mind. Understand that there is no quality control in states where marijuana has not been legalized.

In the event of any legal problems, it's important to know your rights. First, to avoid problems in the first place, never leave your cannabis or paraphernalia in plain view. Second, do not consent to a search. If you consent, you waive your constitutional protection and the officer may search and seize your possessions without further authorization. If they find anything, you can be arrested. If you do not consent, the officer must release or detain you, but the fact that you do not consent does not give the officer grounds to detain you or to obtain a warrant. Third, do not answer any questions without an attorney, even if you are not being arrested. You have the right to remain silent, and you should use that right. Finally, ask the officer if you are being detained or arrested. If you are not, you have the legal right to leave.

If you are arrested, again, do not say anything without your attorney present. Do not resist or become physical; always remain calm and polite. If you need a lawyer, you can visit lawyers.norml.org for a list of attorneys in your area.

Recreational States

In the following states, adults can consume cannabis without facing legal action if they adhere to certain requirements. These requirements are outlined in the tables found in Appendix A: Medical Marijuana Laws by State (page 191).

Alaska	**Oregon**
Colorado	**Washington**
District of Columbia	

These states also have medical marijuana programs, details of which you can find in the next section.

Medical States

There are medical marijuana programs in 23 states, along with the District of Columbia.

Alaska	Minnesota
Arizona	Montana
California	Nevada
Colorado	New Hampshire
Connecticut	New Jersey
Delaware	New Mexico
Hawaii	New York
Illinois	Oregon
Maine	Rhode Island
Maryland	Vermont
Massachusetts	Washington
Michigan	

Each state has its own set of limits regarding possession and cultivation, along with approved conditions for obtaining a medical marijuana card. Each state has unique laws to govern their medical programs, so be sure you know what's allowed in your state. In the tables that appear in

Appendix A (page 191), you can find websites that provide more information on each state's program and how to apply for their medical marijuana card.

Illegal States

While many states have legislation under-way, there are 27 states that have no true medical marijuana programs as of January 2016. Some of them have permitted CBD oil for medical purposes, which is a great first step, but it still falls short. CBD is just one compound, and it isn't as effective on its own as it is with the rest of the plant.[21] If you live in one of the following states and choose to pursue the medicinal use of cannabis, it is important to be aware of the laws and risks involved.

Alabama	North Dakota
Arkansas	Ohio
Florida	Oklahoma
Georgia	Pennsylvania
Idaho	South Carolina
Indiana	South Dakota
Iowa	Tennessee
Kansas	Texas
Kentucky	Utah
Louisiana	Virginia
Mississippi	West Virginia
Missouri	Wisconsin
Nebraska	Wyoming
North Carolina	

For more details about the legal risks, such as the types of offenses charged by each state for marijuana possession, check out the tables in Appendix A (page 191).

A POPULAR NEW PRESCRIPTION

“ *The evidence is overwhelming that marijuana can relieve certain types of pain, nausea, vomiting, and other symptoms caused by such illnesses as multiple sclerosis, cancer, and AIDS—or by the harsh drugs sometimes used to treat them. And it can do so with remarkable safety. Indeed, marijuana is less toxic than many of the drugs that physicians prescribe every day.”*
—**Dr. Joycelyn Elders**, public health administrator, former US surgeon general[22]

Between 1987 and 2014, the percentage of people who believed marijuana to be “morally wrong” fell from 70 percent to 35 percent.[23] This drastic shift in public opinion has been one of the biggest catalysts in the pro-legalization efforts. A 2013 poll found that 77 percent of the overall public believed cannabis to have legitimate medical uses.[24]

Just 10 years ago, cannabis was an underground drug and the primary focus of the Drug Abuse Resistance Education's popular “Just Say No” campaign. There was

21. R. Gallily, Z. Yekhtin, and L. Hanuš, “Overcoming the Bell-Shaped Dose-Response of Cannabidiol by Using Cannabis Extract Enriched in Cannabidiol,” *Pharmacology & Pharmacy* 6 (2015): 75–85. doi:10.4236/pp.2015.62010. **22.** Joycelyn Elders, “Myths About Medical Marijuana,” *The Providence Journal*, March 26, 2004. **23.** “CNN Poll: Support for Legal Marijuana Soaring,” *CNN*, January 6, 2014, politicalticker.blogs.cnn.com/2014/01/06/cnn-poll-support-for-legal-marijuana-soaring. **24.** “Majority Now Supports Legalizing Marijuana,” *Pew Research Center*, April 4, 2013, www.people-press.org/2013/04/04/majority-now-supports-legalizing-marijuana/.

no recognized medicinal use, and it was a prominent target in the war on drugs. While marijuana is still classified as a Schedule I drug and is federally illegal, the states that have instituted a medical or recreational market have created a haven for its use and decriminalized the drug. The approved criteria for medicinal usage differs slightly state by state as presented in the previous section. As new studies emerge, new criteria and conditions are added to the approved list for medical usage. In California alone, 5 percent of the population uses medical marijuana, and that number is continuing to increase.[25]

Current research on marijuana's efficacy is ongoing, and newer, more potent strains continue to be developed. In other words, the marijuana that people smoked in the 1960s is not what you will find on the market today. As investors pour money into this booming market and cultivators experiment with growing techniques and crossbreeding, marijuana continues to change in potency and strength. NORML fiercely scours new publications and research for unbiased, well-run studies, surveys, and experiments that provide new information on marijuana. To keep up to date on all future research and findings, we suggest that you subscribe to NORML's newsletter. You can also check out the list of reputable sources at the end of this book,

as well as the NORML webpage: norml.org /library/recent-research-on-medical -marijuana. Also, consider giving the book *Stoned: A Doctor's Case for Medical Marijuana* by David Casarett, MD, a read.

If you are interested in treating your own condition with medical marijuana, it can be hard to know where to start. Talk to a trusted doctor who knows your healthcare history, if possible. Being able to show an existing doctor–patient relationship and history of a particular condition may be required for your state's medical marijuana program.

If you don't have an existing relationship with a physician, talk with your NORML community for recommendations. Always check if a particular doctor is covered by your health insurance provider. A good physician should be open to hearing about any alternative healthcare treatments you are interested in pursuing. If a physician brushes off your inquiry or denies it for personal reasons, seek a second opinion.

When you want to bring up the subject of cannabis with your doctor, bring your state's medical marijuana guidelines and list of approved medical criteria. Also bring along some research relevant to how medical marijuana can treat your health condition. If you already have your marijuana medical card, check out chapter 3 for practical information about finding dispensaries and figuring out the delivery method that is best for you.

---

25. S. Ryan-Ibarra, M. Induni, and D. Ewing, "Prevalence of Medical Marijuana Use in California, 2012," *Drug and Alcohol Review* 34, no. 2 (March 2015): 141–46, doi:10.1111/dar.12207.

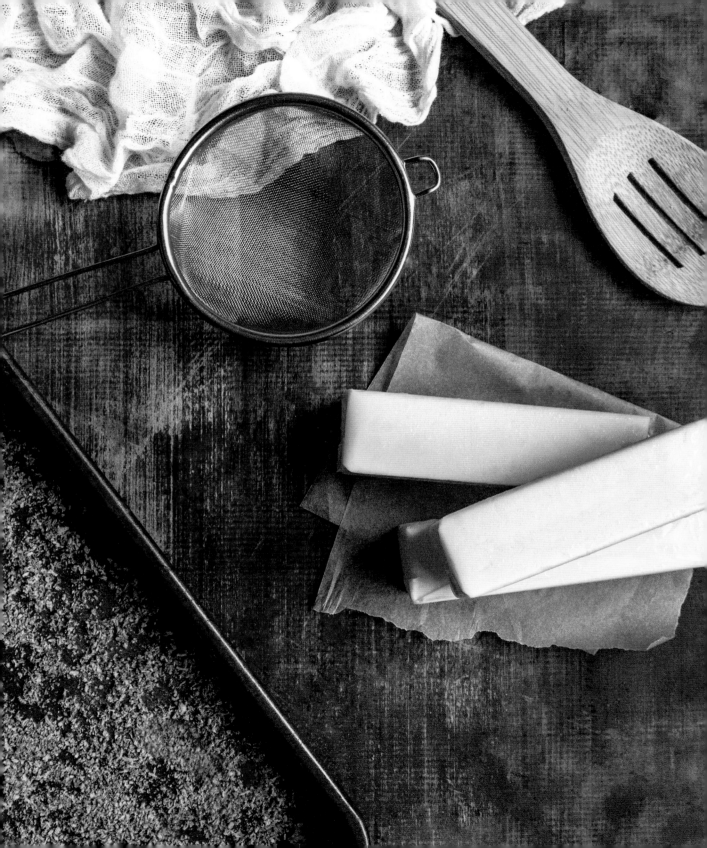

CHAPTER TWO

MARIJUANA AS MEDICINE

THERE IS AN astounding range of health benefits and medicinal treatments offered by marijuana. Cannabis can have antiseizure, anti-inflammatory, antinausea, antianxiety, antidepressant, sedative, neuroprotective, and pain-relieving effects. New research continues to emerge and confirm the efficacy of both modern and centuries-old therapies. Still, it's important to understand the risks involved before medicating with cannabis. Once you find your dosage and delivery method, medical marijuana can provide you with wonderful, much-needed relief.

PROS AND CONS OF MEDICAL MARIJUANA USE

" *I have found in my study of these patients that cannabis is really a safe, effective, and nontoxic alternative to many standard medications. There is no such thing as an overdose. We have seen very minimal problems with abuse or dependence, which at worst are equivalent to dependence on caffeine. While a substance may have some potential for misuse, in my opinion, that's a poor excuse to deny its use and benefit to everyone else."* —**Philip Denney, MD**, physician and cofounder of a medical cannabis evaluation practice

Although the health benefits of marijuana are extremely promising, marijuana is by no means a miracle cure. It is important to continue treatments prescribed by your doctor and not take any rash actions until you are cleared by a knowledgeable physician. Cannabis can certainly help with several symptoms of serious diseases, like multiple sclerosis, epilepsy, and Parkinson's disease, but there is no medical evidence that cannabis can cure any disease. Although scientists are optimistic that marijuana will prove to be helpful in treating many serious illnesses, and perhaps even offer a cure, there is a need for more clinical studies.

Recent research suggests a wide range of clinical applications for cannabis. Studies show it can help combat symptoms like nausea, pain, pressure from glaucoma, inflammation, muscle spasms, headaches and migraines, lack of appetite, sleeplessness, anxiety, and depression. Some studies suggest that it can even stop the spread of cancer cells and slow the progression of Alzheimer's disease; research into these areas is ongoing.

Finding out if cannabis is right for you is a process that takes time. If you have a medical condition that cannabis is reported to help, talk with a medical professional about how to start the process.

Benefits of Using Medical Marijuana versus Other Health Treatments

You can't overdose on cannabis. In marijuana's lengthy history, there has been no record of a fatal overdose (compare that to the 6 people each day who are killed by alcohol poisoning or the 40 people each day who are killed by prescription painkiller overdose).[26]

There are fewer negative side effects. Some prescription drugs have really nasty side effects that can lead to nausea, congestive heart failure, heart attacks, stroke, cancer, physical debilitation, and even death.[27]

The cost is low. Prescriptions can be quite expensive, and while you still have to pay for medical marijuana, it is certainly more affordable than most prescription drugs. With a green thumb and a little setup cost, you can even grow your own medicine.

It helps your metabolism. Recent studies demonstrate a link between cannabis use and a lower percentage of body fat. Results found the rate of obesity and diabetes to be dramatically reduced in cannabis users compared to non-cannabis users.[28]

It protects your brain. Modern science has identified the potential neuroprotective nature of cannabis, especially in relation to alcohol-induced brain damage. In sharp contrast to the belief that marijuana kills brain cells, cannabinoids have, in some instances, been associated with the protection and generation of brain cells.[29]

It can relieve pain. Marijuana can relieve chronic pain, particularly neuropathic pain, which is nerve-associated pain that is notoriously hard to treat with standard analgesics.

You can use it to relax. Cannabis can relax your body and your mind, which is helpful when treating insomnia, anxiety, and PTSD.

It increases appetite. The cannabinoid THC stimulates your appetite, making it great for health conditions that cause a lack of appetite and lead to physical weakness.

It reduces nausea. Along with increasing the appetite, marijuana reduces nausea. Patients who are going through chemotherapy need

26. "National Vital Statistics System: Mortality Data," *Centers for Disease Control and Prevention*, December 30, 2015, www.cdc.gov/nchs/deaths.htm. **27.** "Dangerous Prescription," *PBS Frontline*, November 13, 2003, www.pbs.org/wgbh/pages/frontline/shows/prescription/etc/synopsis.html. **28.** G. Ngueta et al., "Cannabis Use in Relation to Obesity and Insulin Resistance in the Inuit Population," *Obesity* 23, no. 2 (February 2015): 290–95, doi:10.1002/oby.20973. **29.** C. Hamelink, "Comparison of Cannabidiol, Antioxidants, and Diuretics in Reversing Binge Ethanol-Induced Neurotoxicity," *Journal of Pharmacology and Experimental Therapeutics* 314, no. 2 (August 2005): 780–88, www.ncbi.nlm.nih.gov/pubmed/15878999.

to keep their strength up, but eating may be the last thing they want to do. Cannabis can stimulate their appetite by reducing nausea.

Drawbacks of Using Medical Marijuana versus Other Health Treatments

Your thought process and motor coordination can become impaired. High doses of THC may cause impairments to short-term memory, balance, and coordination. Never drive or operate heavy machinery when using cannabis.

You can experience dry mouth. One of the most common side effects of marijuana use is feeling like you have a bunch of cotton balls in your mouth. Keep a drink or ice pop handy!

It can increase your appetite. Cannabis is prescribed for patients with a lack of appetite or nausea, because, well, it increases your appetite. This may not be a welcome side effect, however, if you already have a healthy appetite.

It temporarily increases heart rate. If you have heart issues, talk with your doctor before medicating with cannabis. An increased heart rate may increase your risk of heart attack.

Hallucinations can occur. Cannabis is a mild psychedelic. High doses of THC may cause auditory or visual hallucinations.

You may feel anxiety, distrust, and panic. High doses of cannabis or even moderate doses of some strains may lead to these negative feelings. However, cannabis can also decrease anxiety.

There are unpredictable effects from strain to strain. Different strains may affect you in different ways, and the same strain may be different from one grower to the next.

Inhalation of tar and chemicals can be harmful. Inhaling smoke from cannabis brings harmful tar and chemicals into the lungs and throat. While long-term studies haven't found a correlation between smoking cannabis and lung damage, patients with sensitive or weakened lungs or throat should avoid smoking.

Long-term effects are unclear. Modern research has pointed to a number of wonderful benefits from cannabis, but studies are lacking on the long-term effects of the various methods of cannabis use.

Cannabis use is federally illegal. Cannabis is banned by the federal government. Using it may put you at risk for legal action. Refer to the tables in Appendix A to review your state's marijuana limits.

Not much is known about the effects of mixing prescription drugs and marijuana. In the case of some antidepressants, cannabis can increase undesirable side effects such as anxiety, nausea, and rapid heart rate. With antipsychotics, the very symptoms that are being treated may be made worse with the use of marijuana. Again, there is very little research on the mixing of cannabis with prescription drugs. When in doubt, talk with your doctor.

When Use Becomes Abuse

The jury is still out on the addictive nature of cannabis. Research suggests that the release of the neurotransmitter dopamine can trigger an addiction circuit in the brain similar to that triggered by sugar and alcohol. The feel-good effects of dopamine cause the brain to tell us that it wants more. Just seeing a picture of the substance in question can cause our brain to start firing in anticipation.

One study showed that 40 percent of participants who stopped using cannabis experienced withdrawal symptoms, including insomnia, depression, anxiety, and panic attacks.[30] This is concerning because those are some of the exact conditions cannabis is known to treat. That said, many pharmaceutical drugs are seriously addictive and have highly unpleasant withdrawal symptoms. As with any medicine you take, you must know the potential risks and side effects.

Ask yourself:

☐ Are you becoming too dependent on medical marijuana?

☐ Do you need to smoke more to achieve the same effects?

☐ Have you experienced any withdrawal symptoms when you've tried to stop, such as sleep disturbances or irritability?

☐ Have you tried and failed to stop using cannabis?

☐ Do you spend a significant amount of time trying to obtain, use, or recover from the effects of marijuana?

☐ Have you given up important social or work activities to use cannabis?

☐ Do you continue to use cannabis despite experiencing consistent negative side effects?

If you answered yes to any of the preceding questions, you may need to take a break from medical marijuana for a month. This is known as a tolerance break. Research has shown that 28 days may be sufficient to reset the body's processing of cannabis. If you find you need help stopping, please contact your doctor or therapist.

---

30. M. C. Greene and J. F. Kelly, "The Prevalence of Cannabis Withdrawal and Its Influence on Adolescents' Treatment Response and Outcomes: A 12-Month Prospective Investigation," *Journal of Addiction Medicine* 8, no. 5 (September–October 2014): 359–67. doi:10.1097/ADM.0000000000000064.

CHRONIC CARE FOR CHRONIC HEALTH ISSUES

66 *The American Nurses Association (ANA) recognizes that patients should have safe access to therapeutic marijuana/cannabis. Cannabis or marijuana has been used medicinally for centuries. It has been shown to be effective in treating a wide range of symptoms and conditions."* —**American Nurses Association**

We've used research on medical and therapeutic uses of marijuana and its cannabinoids published in the last 15 years to compile the following list of health conditions that may be treated with cannabis. Remember, cannabis is not a miracle drug, and it is not the answer to all illnesses and maladies. In addition, not everyone will benefit from cannabis in the same way, so anecdotal evidence should be viewed as just that—anecdotal. That being said, cannabis does have an astounding array of clinical applications and health benefits. As new studies continue to emerge, we recommend that you stay current on the research and its published findings. NORML, and particularly the NORML blog at blog.norml.org, is a great source of information on reliable studies as they are released.

Health Issues and Symptoms with Substantial Research

Chronic pain: A study in 2013 found that the inhalation and ingestion of THC significantly decreased pain sensitivity in healthy subjects exposed to pain.[31] Cannabis can also reduce the risk of abuse and overdose associated with pharmaceutical opioids. "States permitting medical marijuana dispensaries experience a relative decrease in both opioid addictions and opioid overdose deaths compared to states that do not," reported the National Bureau of Economic Research.[32] Unfortunately, some states do not include chronic pain as a qualifying condition for medical marijuana.

HIV and AIDS: Cannabis is a very common treatment for patients suffering with HIV or AIDS. Not only does it combat neuropathic pain,[33] nausea, loss of appetite, and anxiety, but it can also improve the immune system of patients living with HIV or AIDS.[34] A 2011 study found an association between cannabis and decreased mortality and reduction in disease progression.[35]

Nausea: The antinausea properties of cannabis are well researched. Cannabis is often prescribed to cancer patients going through

31. Z. D. Cooper et al., "Comparison of the Analgesic Effects of Dronabinol and Smoked Marijuana in Daily Marijuana Smokers," *Neuropsychopharmacology* 38, no. 10 (September 2013): 1984–92, doi:10.1038/npp.2013.97. **32.** David Powell et al., "Do Medical Marijuana Laws Reduce Addictions and Deaths Related to Pain Killers?" NBER Working Paper No. 21345 (July 2015), www.nber.org/papers/w21345. **33.** D. I. Abrams et al., "Cannabis in Painful HIV-Associated Sensory Neuropathy: A Randomized Placebo-Controlled Trial," *Neurology* 68, no. 7 (February 13, 2007): 515–21, www.ncbi.nlm.nih.gov/pubmed/17296917. **34.** A. Fogarty et al., "Marijuana as Therapy for People Living with HIV/AIDS: Social and Health Aspects," *AIDS Care* 19, no. 2 (February 2007): 295–301, www.ncbi.nlm.nih.gov/pubmed/17364413. **35.** P. E. Molina et al., "Cannabinoid Administration Attenuates the Progression of Simian Immunodeficiency Virus," *AIDS Research and Human Retroviruses* 27, no. 6 (June 2011): 585–92, doi:10.1089/AID.2010.0218.

chemotherapy as a remedy for nausea and an appetite stimulant.[36]

Neuropathic pain: Chronic nerve pain is often associated with cancer, HIV or AIDS, spinal cord injury, and diabetes. Several studies have found that cannabis treats this pain better than currently available medications.[37]

Multiple sclerosis (MS): Studies show that marijuana reduces many symptoms of multiple sclerosis, including depression, fatigue, incontinence, spasticity, and pain.[38] Research is now focusing on the ability of cannabinoids to modify the disease itself. A 2003 study suggests that the neuroprotective properties of cannabis may "slow the neurodegenerative processes that ultimately lead to chronic disability in multiple sclerosis."[39]

Rheumatoid arthritis: Cannabis has been shown to relieve the pain and inflammation of rheumatoid arthritis, as well as the progression of the disease itself.[40]

Health Issues and Symptoms with a Moderate Amount of Research

Amyotrophic lateral sclerosis (ALS): Preclinical data shows the ability of cannabinoids to halt the progression of ALS and relieve certain symptoms and side effects of the disease such as pain, loss of appetite, and depression.[41] The scientific community is calling for clinical trials to validate these findings and move forward in the treatment of the disease with cannabis.

Alzheimer's disease: As a study in 2006 found, "THC and its analogues may provide an improved therapeutic [option] for Alzheimer's disease [by] . . . simultaneously treating both the symptoms and the progression of [the] disease."[42] Additional studies show weight gain and a decrease in negative feelings to also be positive effects of cannabinoids on Alzheimer's patients.[43]

Acute head trauma: Cannabinoids have been shown to act as a neuroprotectant in a 2013

36. Barliz Waissengrin et al., "Patterns of Use of Medical Cannabis Among Israeli Cancer Patients: A Single Institution Experience," *Journal of Pain and Symptom Management* 49, no. 2 (February 2015): 223–30, doi:10.1016/j.jpainsymman.2014.05.018. **37.** Darrell G. Boychuk et al., "The Effectiveness of Cannabinoids in the Management of Chronic Nonmalignant Neuropathic Pain: A Systematic Review," *Journal of Oral & Facial Pain and Headache* 29, no. 1 (2015): 7–14, doi:10.11607/ofph.1274. **38.** Jody Corey-Bloom, "Short-Term Effects of Cannabis Therapy on Spasticity in Multiple Sclerosis." In: University of San Diego Health Sciences, Center for Medicinal Cannabis Research. *Report to the Legislature and Governor of the State of California presenting findings pursuant to SB847 which created the CMCR and provided state funding* (2010). **39.** Gareth Pryce et al., "Cannabinoids Inhibit Neurodegeneration in Models of Multiple Sclerosis," *Brain* 126 (July 2003): 2191–202. **40.** D. R. Blake et al., "Preliminary Assessment of the Efficacy, Tolerability and Safety of a Cannabis Medicine (Sativex) in the Treatment of Pain Caused by Rheumatoid Arthritis," *Rheumatology* 45, no. 1 (January 2006): 50–52, www.ncbi.nlm.nih.gov/pubmed/16282192. **41.** D. Amtmann et al., "Survey of Cannabis Use in Patients with Amyotrophic Lateral Sclerosis," *The American Journal of Hospice and Palliative Care* 21, no. 2 (March–April 2004): 95–104, www.ncbi.nlm.nih.gov/pubmed/15055508. **42.** Lisa M. Eubanks et al., "A Molecular Link Between the Active Component of Marijuana and Alzheimer's Disease Pathology," *Molecular Pharmaceutics* 3, no. 6 (2006): 773–77, doi:10.1021/mp060066m. **43.** "Cannabis Lifts Alzheimer's Appetite," *BBC News*, August 21, 2003.

study, protecting the brain from damage before and after an injury.[44]

Stroke: A 2015 meta-analysis found cannabinoids to significantly reduce the injury from stroke and improve the functional outcomes of stroke victims when administered 2 to 6 hours after the stroke.[45]

Parkinson's disease: A recent 2014 study reported significant improvements in the Parkinson's disease symptoms of tremors, rigidity, and slowness of movement.[46] Daily use also corresponded to improved sleep, quality of life, and overall well-being.[47]

Diabetes: Several studies indicated an inverse relationship between cannabis use and diabetes.[48] Cannabinoids are shown to halt disease progression,[49] resist disease development,[50] and treat side effects of those with the disease such as diabetic retinopathy[51] (the leading cause of blindness in adults) and neuropathic pain.[52] In a recent study, subjects who used cannabis in the past year were more likely to have a lower percentage of body fat, lower waist circumference, and lower insulin resistance compared to those who had not reported use of the substance.[53]

Epilepsy: While reports of treating epilepsy, a nervous system disorder that causes twitching and seizures, with cannabis are numerous, especially in pediatric patients, clinical studies are only now being conducted.[54] Recent research focusing on CBD as a treatment for the disorder are finding a decrease in the frequency of seizures for pediatric patients.[55]

---

44. M. Fishbein et al., "Long-Term Behavioral and Biochemical Effects of an Ultra-Low Dose of Δ9-Tetrahydrocannabinol (THC): Neuroprotection and ERK Signaling," *Experimental Brain Research* 221, no. 4 (September 2012): 437–48. doi:10.1007/s00221-012-3186-5. **45.** T. J. England et al., "Cannabinoids in Experimental Stroke: A Systematic Review and Meta-Analysis." *Journal of Cerebral Blood Flow & Metabolism* 35, no. 3 (March 2015): 348–58, doi:10.1038/jcbfm.2014.218. **46.** I. Lotan et al., "Cannabis (Medical Marijuana) Treatment for Motor and Non-Motor Symptoms of Parkinson Disease: An Open-Label Observational Study," *Clinical Neuropharmacology* 37, no. 2 (March–April 2014): 41–44. doi:10.1097/WNF.0000000000000016. **47.** M. H. Chagas et al., "Effects of Cannabidiol in the Treatment of Patients with Parkinson's Disease: An Exploratory Double-Blind Trial," *Journal of Psychopharmacology* 28, no. 11 (November 2014): 1088–98. doi:10.1177/0269881114550355. **48.** O. Alshaarway and J. C. Anthony, "Cannabis Smoking and Diabetes Mellitus: Results from Meta-Analysis with Eight Independent Replication Samples," *Epidemiology* 26, no. 4 (July 2015): 597–600, doi:10.1097/EDE.0000000000000314. **49.** E. T. Wargent et al., "The Cannabinoid Δ9-Tetrahydrocannabivarin (THCV) Ameliorates Insulin Sensitivity in Two Mouse Models of Obesity," *Nutrition & Diabetes* 3 (May 27, 2013): e68, doi:10.1038/nutd.2013.9. **50.** L. Weiss et al., "Cannabidiol Lowers Incidence of Diabetes in Non-Obese Diabetic Mice," *Autoimmunity* 39, no. 2 (March 2006): 143–51, www.ncbi.nlm.nih.gov/pubmed/16698671. **51.** A. B. El-Remessy et al., "Neuroprotective and Blood-Retinal Barrier Preserving Effects of Cannabidiol in Experimental Diabetes," *American Journal of Pathology* 168, no. 1 (January 2006), 235–44, www.ncbi.nlm.nih.gov/pubmed/16400026. **52.** M. S. Wallace et al., "Efficacy of Inhaled Cannabis on Painful Diabetic Neuropathy," *The Journal of Pain* 16, no. 7 (July 2015), 616–27. doi:10.1016/j.jpain.2015.03.008. **53.** G. Ngueta et al., "Cannabis Use in Relation to Obesity and Insulin Resistance in the Inuit Population," *Obesity*, 23, no. 2 (February 2015), 290–95, doi:10.1002/oby.20973. **54.** J. I. Sirven, "Marijuana for Epilepsy: Winds of Change," *Epilepsy & Behavior* 29, no. 3 (December 2013): 435–36. doi:10.1016/j.yebeh.2013.09.004. **55.** "Medical Marijuana Liquid Extract May Bring Hope for Children with Severe Epilepsy," *American Academy of Neurology*, April 13, 2015, www.aan.com/PressRoom/home/PressRelease/1364.

Fibromyalgia: Patients suffering from fibromyalgia have few working options for treating their chronic pain. While there have only been a few medical trials investigating the use of cannabis for the treatment of fibromyalgia, many patients are praising its efficacy.[56] In 2011, a study found that fibromyalgia patients successfully used cannabis to treat pain and stiffness and to promote relaxation.[57]

Gastrointestinal disorders: Patients with gastrointestinal disorders, such as irritable bowel syndrome (IBS), Crohn's disease, and inflammatory bowel disease (IBD), often find relief with cannabis. Studies show that cannabis can improve symptoms by suppressing gastrointestinal motility,[58] inhibiting intestinal secretions,[59] reducing acid reflux,[60] and protecting from inflammation,[61] as well as promoting epithelial wound healing.[62]

Cancer/glioma (brain and spinal cord tumor): A growing body of preclinical and clinical data demonstrates the ability of cannabinoids to reduce the spread of specific cancer cells and to possibly even kill those cells. These promising findings are providing hope for a new class of cancer treatment using cannabis.[63] For up-to-date information, visit the National Cancer Institute's page on cannabis treatment (see Resources on page 205).

Urinary incontinence: Patients with multiple sclerosis and spinal cord injuries found relief from incontinence with cannabis in a 2003 study.[64] Experts believe there may be broader applications for the wider population suffering with incontinence.[65]

Methicillin-resistant *Staphylococcus aureus* **(MRSA):** The antibacterial properties of cannabis have demonstrated great success in reducing the spread of the multidrug-resistant bacterial infection MRSA in preclinical models.[66]

Posttraumatic stress disorder (PTSD): Experts believe that cannabis can ease

56. "Marijuana Rated Most Effective for Treating Fibromyalgia," *National Pain Report*, April 21, 2014, nationalpainreport.com /marijuana-rated-most-effective-for-treating-fibromyalgia-8823638.html. **57.** Jimena Fiz et al., "Cannabis Use in Patients with Fibromyalgia: Effect on Symptoms Relief and Health-Related Quality of Life," *PLoS One* 6, no. 4 (April 2011), e18440, doi:10.1371/journal .pone.0018440. **58.** Roger G. Pertwee, "Cannabinoids and the Gastrointestinal Tract," *Gut* 48, no. 6 (June 2001), 859–67, www.ncbi .nlm.nih.gov/pubmed/11358910. **59.** G. Di Carlo and A. A. Izzo, "Cannabinoids for Gastrointestinal Diseases: Potential Therapeutic Applications," *Expert Opinion on Investigational Drugs*, 12 no. 1 (January 2003), 39–49, www.ncbi.nlm.nih.gov/pubmed/12517253. **60.** A. Lehmann et al., "Cannabinoid Receptor Agonism Inhibits Transient Lower Esophageal Sphincter Relaxations and Reflux in Dogs." *Gastroenterology* 123, no. 4 (October 2002), 1129–34, www.ncbi.nlm.nih.gov/pubmed/12360475. **61.** Massa et al., "The Endo-cannabinoid System in the Physiology and Pathophysiology of the Gastrointestinal Tract." *Journal of Molecular Medicine* 12, no. 1 (2005): 944–54. **62.** K. Wright et al., "Differential Expression of Cannabinoid Receptors in the Human Colon: Cannabinoids Promote Epithelial Wound Healing," *Gastroenterology* 129, no. 2 (August 2005): 437–53, www.ncbi.nlm.nih.gov/pubmed/16083701. **63.** Sami Sarafaraz et al., "Cannabinoids for Cancer Treatment: Progress and Promise," *Cancer Research* 68 (January 2008): 339–42. doi:10.1158/0008-5472.CAN-07-2785. **64.** D. T. Wade et al., "A Preliminary Controlled Study to Determine Whether Whole-Plant Cannabis Extracts Can Improve Intractable Neurogenic Symptoms," *Clinical Rehabilitation* 17, no. 1 (February 2003): 21–29, www.ncbi .nlm.nih.gov/pubmed/12617376. **65.** "Marijuana-Derived Drug Suppresses Bladder Pain in Animal Models," *University of Pittsburgh Medical Center*, May 21, 2006. **66.** Giovanni Appendino et al., "Antibacterial Cannabinoids from Cannabis Sativa: A Structure Study," *Journal of Natural Products* 71, no. 8 (August 2008): 1427–30. doi:10.1021/np8002673.

symptoms of PTSD by relieving anxiety, depression, and insomnia.[67]

Pruritus (itching): Patients medicating with cannabis saw a decrease in their chronic itching and were able to sleep better and return to work.[68] Topical application cured pruritus in 38 percent of trial subjects in a 2005 study and significantly reduced the itching in another 43 percent.[69]

Tourette syndrome: Clinical studies report a significant reduction of tics and obsessive-compulsive behavior associated with Tourette syndrome in patients who were given THC.[70]

Health Issues and Symptoms that Need More Research

Alcohol-induced brain damage: A 2005 study on rats demonstrated a 60 percent reduction in brain cell death caused by ethanol abuse with the help of the cannabinoid CBD.[71]

Depression and anxiety: Research suggests that cannabinoids can play a role in the alleviation of depression and anxiety and that cannabis-based medicines may one day offer a safer alternative to conventional antidepressant pharmaceuticals.[72]

Hepatitis C: Existing treatments for hepatitis C can often cause nausea. Cannabis can treat not only the nausea but also the symptoms of the disease (depression, fatigue, joint pain, and cirrhosis).[73] More research is needed to properly assess the safety of cannabis for this disease, as a recent study found a link between cannabis and steatosis (fatty liver) in hepatitis C patients.[74]

Dystonia (involuntary muscle contractions): Several case studies have been published on the successful treatment of dystonia, a neurological movement disorder causing muscle tension and contractions, with cannabis. One study reported the patient's subjective pain score fell from 9 (out of 10) to 0 for 48 hours after inhaling marijuana.[75] Other reports found improvement in motor control and a possible halt in the progression of the

67. T. Passie et al., "Mitigation of Post-Traumatic Stress Symptoms by Cannabis Resin: A Review of the Clinical and Neurobiological Evidence," *Drug Testing and Analysis* 4, no. 7–8 (July–August 2012): 649–59. doi:10.1002/dta.1377. **68.** J. W. Neff et al., "Preliminary Observation with Dronabinol in Patients with Intractable Pruritus Secondary to Cholestatic Liver Disease," *American Journal of Gastroenterology* 97, no. 8 (August 2002): 2117–19, www.ncbi.nlm.nih.gov/pubmed/12190187. **69.** J. C. Szepietowski et al., "Efficacy and Tolerance of the Cream Containing Structured Physiological Lipid Endocannabinoids in the Treatment of Uremic Pruritus: A Preliminary Study." *Acta Dermatovenerologic Croatica* 13, no. 2 (2005): 97–103, www.ncbi.nlm.nih.gov/pubmed/16324422. **70.** Kirsten R. Müller-Vahl, "Treatment of Tourette's Syndrome with Delta-9-tetrahydrocannabinol (THC): A Randomized Crossover Trial," *Pharmacopsychiatry* 35 (2002): 57–61. doi:10.3233/BEN-120276. **71.** Carol Hamelink et al., "Comparison of Cannabidiol, Antioxidants and Diuretics in Reversing Binge Ethanol-Induced Neurotoxicity," *Journal of Pharmacology and Experimental Therapeutics* 314, no. 2 (August 2005): 780–88, accessed January 2, 2016, www.ncbi.nlm.nih.gov/pubmed/15878999. **72.** Wen Jiang et al., "Cannabinoids Promote Embryonic and Adult Hippocampus Neurogenesis and Produce Anxiolytic and Antidepressant-like Effects," *The Journal of Clinical Investigation* 115, no. 11 (2005): 3104–16. doi:10.1172/JCI25509. **73.** David Bernstein, "Hepatitis C—Current State of the Art and Future Directions," *MedScape Gastroenterology,* December 8, 2004, www.medscape.com/viewarticle/495211. **74.** V. Purohit et al., "Role of Cannabinoids in the Development of Fatty Liver (Steatosis)," *The AAPS Journal* 12, no. 2 (June 2010): 233–7. doi:10.1208/s12248-010-9178-0. **75.** A. Chatterjee et al., "A Dramatic Response to Inhaled Cannabis in a Woman with Central Thalamic Pain and Dystonia," *The Journal of Pain and Symptom Management* 24, no. 1 (July 2002): 4–6, doi:http://dx.doi.org/10.1016/S0885-3924(02)00426-8.

disease.[76] Larger clinical trials are warranted to investigate this treatment across the population suffering from dystonia.

Hypertension (high blood pressure): Experts believe there is a strong link between the endocannabinoid system (a group of body-wide cannabinoid receptors) and the regulation of blood pressure.[77] Animal studies have demonstrated a link between cannabis and lowering blood pressure, as well as reducing the progression of the hardening of arteries.[78] Human clinical trials are needed to assess the efficacy of cannabis in lowering blood pressure.

Huntington's disease: While cannabis has not been shown to relieve symptoms of Huntington's disease, a brain nerve cell disorder, it may play a role in moderating the advancement of the disease. A combination of THC and CBD has neuroprotective properties that may delay disease progression.[79]

Osteoporosis: Scientists believe that the primary role of some endocannabinoid receptors is to keep "bone remodeling at balance, thus protecting the skeleton against age-related bone loss," which has

caused some experts to speculate that marijuana may be a possible treatment for osteoporosis.[80]

Sleep apnea: Animal studies report a significant reduction of sleep-related apnea with cannabis use. Researchers found that properties in cannabis help stabilize respiration during sleep and block serotonin-induced exacerbation of sleep apnea in a statistically significant manner.[81]

Separating Fact from Fiction

As you continue on your cannabis journey, you may encounter naysayers who will list several dangers of cannabis. While there are very real risks (covered earlier in this chapter), we'll lay out some facts for you now.

- There are no reports that anyone has ever overdosed or died from smoking or consuming too much cannabis.

- A 2012 study on cannabis's effects on the lungs found that occasional and low cannabis use caused no adverse effects.[82] In fact, the anti-inflammatory properties of cannabis can potentially benefit both asthma and lung functioning.

76. A. Richter and W. Löscher, "Effects of Pharmacological Manipulations of Cannabinoid Receptors on Severe Dystonia in a Genetic Model of Paroxysmal Dyskinesia," *European Journal of Pharmacology* 454, no. 2-3 (November 2002): 145–51, www.ncbi.nlm.nih.gov/pubmed/12421641. **77.** P. Pacher et al., "Blood Pressure Regulation by Endocannabinoids and Their Receptors," *Neuropharmacology* 48, no. 8 (June 2005): 1130–38, doi:10.1016/j.neuropharm.2004.12.005. **78.** Steven Karch, "Cannabis and Cardiotoxicity," *Forensic Science, Medicine, and Pathology* 2, (2006): 13–18. **79.** O. Sagredo et al., "Neuroprotective Effects of Phytocannabinoid-Based Medicines in Experimental Models of Huntington's Disease," *Journal of Neuroscience Research* 89, no. 9 (September 2011): 1509–18. doi:10.1002/jnr.22682. **80.** I. Bab et al., "Cannabinoids and the Skeleton: From Marijuana to Reversal of Bone Loss," *Annals of Medicine* 41, no. 8 (2009): 560–67. doi:10.1080/07853890903121025. **81.** D. W. Carley et al., "Functional Role for Cannabinoids in Respiratory Stability During Sleep," *Sleep* 25, no. 4 (June 2002): 391–98, www.ncbi.nlm.nih.gov/pubmed/12071539. **82.** M. J. Pletcher et al., "Association Between Marijuana Exposure and Pulmonary Function Over 20 Years," *The Journal of American Medical Association* 307, no. 2 (January 2012):173–81. doi:10.1001/jama.2011.1961.

- Marijuana is not a gateway drug that may lead to the use of addictive drugs. A 2014 study found that although cannabis use went up in teenagers, hard drug use did not.[83]

- Cannabis use during pregnancy has not been linked to birth defects.[84] (Nevertheless, it is best to avoid it during pregnancy.)

- Cannabis does not kill brain cells. It actually has neuroprotective and neurogenerative properties.[85]

- Cannabis use is less dangerous than drinking alcohol and using tobacco.[86]

To begin medicating with cannabis, start slow. Talk with your doctor about possible drug interactions and any potential health risks. You can also refer to a list of interactions online at www.drugs.com /drug-interactions/cannabis-index.html. If possible, work with a local dispensary to find strains and products that will work best for you and your condition.

Whether inhaling or ingesting, start with very small quantities in a safe place. For edibles, start with products containing 2.5 mg of THC and wait a day before increasing your dosage. For inhalation, start with two small puffs and wait 30 minutes before increasing. Arrange to have someone you can call in case of a negative reaction. Until you know how your body will react, be conservative.

CANNABIS AND THE HUMAN BODY

" *There were never so many able, active minds at work on the problems of disease as now, and all their discoveries are tending toward the simple truth that you can't improve on nature.*" —**Thomas Edison**, inventor and businessman

To explain how cannabis affects the human body, we must first start with an overview of the endocannabinoid system, which was named for the plant that led to its discovery. The recent discovery of this body-wide group of receptors upon which cannabinoids act has exponentially progressed our understanding of marijuana's regulatory functions in health and disease.

Endocannabinoid receptors are found throughout the human body: in the brain, organs, central and peripheral nervous system, cardiovascular system, reproductive system, gastrointestinal system, urinary system, immune system, and even cartilage. The medical community believes that our endocannabinoid system is responsible for regulating the homeostasis of our biological functions, and may subsequently be the most important system in the human body.

Researchers have discovered two cannabinoid receptors, CB1 and CB2. They believe

---

83. "In Nationwide Survey, More Students Use Marijuana, Fewer Use Other Drugs," *National Institute on Drug Abuse,* April 22, 2014, www.drugabuse.gov/news-events/nida-notes/2014/04/in-nationwide-survey-more-students-use-marijuana-fewer-use-other -drugs. **84.** M. C. Dreher et al., "Prenatal Marijuana Exposure and Neonatal Outcomes in Jamaica: An Ethnographic Study," *Pediatrics* 93, no. 2 (February 1994): 254–60, www.ncbi.nlm.nih.gov/pubmed/8121737. **85.** Samuel J. Jackson et al., "Cannabinoids and Neuro-protection in CNS Inflammatory Disease," *Journal of the Neurological Sciences* 233, no. 1–2 (June 2005): 21–25, www.ncbi.nlm.nih .gov/pubmed/15894331. **86.** Wayne Hall, *A Comparative Appraisal of the Health and Psychological Consequences of Alcohol, Cannabis, Nicotine, and Opiate Use* (University of New South Wales: National Drug and Alcohol Research Centre, 1995).

there is a third awaiting discovery. CB1 receptors are found predominantly in our central and peripheral nervous system and CB2 receptors are found in the immune system. Many tissues contain both receptors, each performing distinct actions.[87] Medical studies have found an unusual abundance of cannabinoid receptors in tumor cells. Autophagy, or cell self-deconstruction, is facilitated by the endocannabinoid system, which keeps normal, healthy cells alive while instructing malignant, cancerous cells to self-destruct. Experts believe that the presence of cannabinoid receptors in tumor cells is a clear example of the endocannabinoid system's vital role in our internal homeostasis. Moreover, clinical studies and research show that endocannabinoid deficiencies—that is, a deficiency in the biochemical compounds that activate the same receptors as cannabis—play a role in several medical conditions, including migraines, fibromyalgia, and irritable bowel syndrome (IBS).[88]

To clarify, our bodies naturally make endocannabinoids to stimulate the cannabinoid receptors and regulate the system. Cannabinoids, such as THC, are *external* substances that stimulate those same receptors. Research indicates that the administration of external cannabinoids, such as THC, can cause the endocannabinoid system to create more receptors, and thus increase a patient's sensitivity to the cannabinoids. First-time users might not feel the experience as intensely as they will after a few uses.

THC and other cannabinoids are produced inside the marijuana plant's trichomes and are excreted in the resin. The resin is made up of a mixture of more than 700 chemicals, the most important of which are cannabinoids and terpenes.

THC is the cannabinoid that gets the most attention, and with good reason. It's responsible for the psychoactive effects of marijuana, but it's also helpful for relieving pain, nausea, lack of appetite, and inflammation. THC mimics the cannabinoids naturally produced in the body and activates receptors in the brain associated with thinking, pain, pleasure, time perception, coordination, and concentration.

The second most common cannabinoid, cannabidiol (CBD), acts on different pathways in the brain than THC, so there are little, if any, psychotropic results. CBD possesses anticonvulsant activity, helps with inflammation, has been shown to reduce some tumors and cancer cells, and relieves anxiety and depression disorders. CBD has also been shown to reduce the psychotropic effects of THC, which in large quantities, can be very unpleasant. A study from the 1970s found that patients reported greater relief

---

87. P. Pacher et al., "The Endocannabinoid System as an Emerging Target of Pharmacotherapy." *Pharmacological Reviews* 58, no. 3 (September 2006): 389–462, www.ncbi.nlm.nih.gov/pubmed/16968947. **88.** S. C. Smith and M. S. Wagner, "Clinical Endocannabinoid Deficiency (CECD) Revisited: Can This Concept Explain the Therapeutic Benefits of Cannabis in Migraine, Fibromyalgia, Irritable Bowel Syndrome and Other Treatment-Resistant Conditions?" *Neuro Endocrinology Letters* 35, no. 3 (2014): 198–201, www.ncbi.nlm.nih.gov/pubmed/24977967.

Children and Medical Marijuana

Medicating a child with marijuana can be an alarming thought. No one wants to break the law or give their children a controlled substance that hasn't been approved for their use. Nevertheless, there are some children with epilepsy who don't respond to any existing therapies. The use of cannabis in treating children has grown rapidly following Dr. Sanjay Gupta's CNN special called *Weed*. In this special, Dr. Gupta introduced us to Charlotte Figi, a young girl with epilepsy whose parents were successfully treating her with high-CBD cannabis oil.

Parents are also finding cannabis to be an integral part of cancer treatment for their children, not only to treat the nausea and pain that are side effects of chemotherapy, but also to fight the cancer itself. Some parents who are desperate to pursue medical marijuana as a viable option have moved to states where marijuana has been legalized. This option is certainly not possible for everyone. Other parents travel to neighboring states to obtain cannabis or ask friends or family in legal states to send them supplies.

There is a lack of medical trials involving the use of marijuana in pediatric patients, and its long-term effects have not been studied. Parents should talk with trusted doctors and medical staff to figure out the best treatment option for their children who might benefit from medical marijuana.

from a combination of CBD and THC than THC alone.[89]

When choosing a cannabis strain for your personal medical use, it's helpful to look at the ratio of THC to CBD. Some patients who need CBD find that a 1:1 ratio of THC to CBD is best, while others look for a 1:20 ratio of THC to CBD for a mostly CBD strain.

You may notice distinct aromas from various strains of cannabis. The signature smell and taste of different strains come from the terpenes in the plant resin. As you learned earlier, terpenes are not only found in cannabis; they are present in many of our everyday foods, flowers, and herbs, including black pepper and rosemary. Emerging research has discovered that terpenes work synergistically with cannabinoids to contribute to the overall effect of a strain. Researchers have termed this the "entourage effect."[90] In trying to develop cannabinoid-based drugs, pharmaceutical companies found that whole plant extracts worked better than isolated compounds.[91]

Terpenes have a wide range of effects comparable to the prized medicinal uses

89. I. G. Karniol et al., "Cannabidiol Interferes with the Effects of Delta 9-Tetrahydrocannabinol in Man," *European Journal of Pharmacology* 28, no. 1 (September 1974):172–77, www.ncbi.nlm.nih.gov/pubmed/4609777. **90.** Shimon Ben-Shabat, "An Entourage Effect: Inactive Endogenous Fatty Acid Glycerol Esters Enhance 2-arachidonoyl-glycerol Cannabinoid Activity." *European Journal of Pharmacology* 353, no. 1 (July 1998): 23–31. **91.** Jerome P. Kassirer, "Federal Foolishness and Marijuana," *New England Journal of Medicine* 336, no. 5 (January 1997): 366–67. doi:10.1056/NEJM199701303360509.

TOP CANNABINOIDS

Description	Conditions Treated	Where to Find It
THC Tetrahydrocannabinol (THC) has both psychotropic and medicinal effects. It has anti-inflammatory and antioxidant properties. It binds to cannabinoid receptors in the central nervous system and the immune system, resulting in relaxation, reduced pain, and increased appetite. It appears to protect the brain by reducing inflammation and stimulating neurogenesis.	AIDS, HIV, ALS, Alzheimer's disease, anxiety, arthritis, cancer, Crohn's disease, chronic pain, fibromyalgia, glaucoma, lack of appetite, nausea, neuropathic pain, Huntington's disease, incontinence, insomnia, multiple sclerosis, pruritus, sleep apnea, and Tourette syndrome	It is hard *not* to find THC in cannabis products. Most strains are predominantly THCA, which is converted into THC when heated. Strains will list the THC percentage of the plant. Edibles, tinctures, and concentrates will likely list the milligrams of THC contained in the product.
THCA Raw cannabis contains mostly tetrahydrocannabinolic acid (THCA). Once heated, THCA becomes THC. THCA is nonpsychoactive. It has anti-proliferative and anti-inflammatory abilities, and appears to help chronic immune system disorders.	Arthritis, cancer, endometriosis, lupus, menstrual cramps, muscle spasms, and seizures	Every high-THC strain that has not been heated contains THCA. Raw plants can be juiced for THCA. Unheated tinctures can also be made with high levels of THCA.
THCV Tetrahydrocannabivarin (THCV) is psychoactive, euphoric, and has stronger, faster "high" effects than THC. It is also an appetite suppressant.	Pain and appetite suppressant	The following strains are generally high in THCV levels: Durban Poison and Blue Dream.
CBD Cannabidiol (CBD) is nonpsychoactive and is reported to be anticonvulsive, antipsychotic, antinausea, sedating, and relaxing. It has also been shown to reduce the psychoactive effects and short-term memory loss associated with THC.	Acne, ADHD, Alzheimer's disease, anxiety, arthritis, cancer, chronic pain, depression, diabetes, Dravet syndrome, epilepsy, glaucoma, Huntington's disease, inflammation, mood disorders, multiple sclerosis, neuropathic pain, Parkinson's disease, and schizophrenia	The following strains are generally high in CBD levels: Charlotte's Web, ACDC, Harlequin, Harle-Tsu, Sour Tsunami, Island Sweet Skunk, and Cannatonic.

Description	Conditions Treated	Where to Find It
CBDV Cannabidivarin (CBDV) is nonpsychoactive and has anticonvulsive effects.	Epilepsy	Strains likely to contain CBDV include Harlequin and Island Sweet Skunk.
CBN Cannabinol (CBN) is created when THC is exposed to light and oxygen. It can cause an intense body high, and make users dizzy or groggy. It has mild psychoactive effects and appears to increase the effects of THC. It has medicinal effects, including improving symptoms of epilepsy, reducing muscle spasm, relieving intraocular pressure, and reducing depression.	Depression, epilepsy, glaucoma, inflammation, insomnia, intraocular pressure, muscle spasms, and pain	All strains can produce CBN when exposed to light and oxygen. It may also be possible to find CBN-specific products at your local dispensary.
CBG Cannabigerol (CBG) is nonpsychoactive and is responsible for the production of both THC and CBD. It has sleep-inducing, antimicrobial, antioxidant, and anti-inflammatory properties. It can lower intraocular pressure.	Glaucoma, inflammatory bowel disease, insomnia, and intraocular pressure	Plants that are harvested three-quarters of the way through their cycle may preserve some CBG. Strains that are high in CBG (around 1 percent) include Harlequin.
CBC Cannabichromene (CBC) is nonpsychoactive and has anti-inflammatory, antifungal, and antiviral properties and may contribute to the overall pain-relieving properties of cannabis. It may also inhibit the growth of cancerous cells and stimulate bone growth. It works best in conjunction with CBD and THC.	Depression, inflammation, migraines, neurodegenerative diseases, and pain	While there are no well-known high-CBC strains, the cannabinoid is quickly gaining popularity. Keep a lookout at your local dispensary for emerging CBC products and strains.

TOP TERPENES

Aroma	Other Sources	Effect	Where to Find It
LINALOOL Floral, citrus notes, candy-like	Lavender, citrus, rosewood, coriander	Antipsychotic, antiepileptic, antianxiety, antiacne, sedative, pain reliever, antidepressant	G-13, LA Confidential
CARYOPHYLLENE Rich, peppery, spicy, woody	Thai basil, cloves, black pepper, cotton	Antiseptic, antibacterial, anti-fungal, anti-inflammatory; good for arthritis, ulcers, autoimmune disorders, and other gastrointestinal complications	Hash Plant, Super Silver Haze
MYRCENE Musky, earthy, herbal with notes of citrus and tropical fruit	Mango, hops, bay leaves, lemongrass, eucalyptus	Sedating, relaxing, pain-relieving, antispasm, anti-inflammatory, anti-insomnia	White Widow, Harlequin
LIMONENE Bitter, sour, citrus	Citrus rind, rosemary, juniper, peppermint	Elevated mood, stress relief, antifungal, antibacterial, anti-carcinogenic; fights gastric reflux, gastrointestinal issues, gallstones, depression, and anxiety	O.G. Kush, Super Lemon Haze
PINENE Sweet, pine	Pine, rosemary, basil, parsley, dill	Asthma, inflammation, alertness, memory retention; may counteract THC effects	Jack Herer, Chemdawg, Bubba Kush, Trainwreck, Super Silver Haze
TERPINOLENE Woody, smoky	Apples, cumin, tea tree, lilacs, conifers	Antifungal, antibacterial, anti-insomnia, antioxidant, anticarcinogenic, sedative	Super Lemon Haze, Jack Herer

of cannabinoids, including pain-relieving, antianxiety, anti-inflammatory, and anti-epileptic effects. Gone are the days of judging a strain by its THC percentage and *indica* versus *sativa*. Testing facilities and dispensaries are now often equipped with the cannabinoid and terpene profile to narrow in on a strain that will work for your unique purpose. Understanding the differences between terpenes will turn you into a true "cannasseur."

When cannabis is inhaled, the chemical compounds travel into the airway and lungs before being absorbed into the bloodstream. Heating the plant during inhalation converts the cannabinoid THCA into the psychoactive compound THC (delta-9 THC), a process known as decarboxylation. As much as 50 to 60 percent of the THC is delivered into the bloodstream, with peak concentrations reached at 5 to 10 minutes after inhalation. Within minutes of inhaling cannabis, the heart rate increases by 20 to 50 beats per minute and can continue for up to 3 hours. The effects of cannabis begin somewhere between 30 seconds to 2 minutes after inhalation, once the drug travels up the bloodstream to the brain, and can last 1 to 2 hours.

If cannabis is consumed in food or drink, the drug will be processed in the stomach before heading to the liver, where much of the THC is converted into a substance necessary for metabolism, the metabolite 11-hydroxy-delta-9-THC. This crosses the blood–brain barrier more easily and is thought to have more of a psychotropic effect than standard THC. It may take anywhere from 30 minutes to 2 hours for effects to kick in, and they can last 4 to 8 hours. There are multiple factors that contribute to how quickly you begin to feel effects. For example, consuming cannabis on an empty stomach can bring on the effects faster than a full stomach, as can a faster metabolism.

On the other hand, hard candies, gum, tincture drops that are administered under the tongue, and anything else absorbed in the mouth will take effect almost immediately and wear off within 2 to 3 hours. Drinks, chocolates, and other edibles can also be absorbed orally to some degree, depending on the length of time the infused product remains in the mouth.

Cannabis suppositories are another efficient and fast way to medicate without inhalation or ingestion. They are shaped like bullets and administered rectally. The chemical compounds are absorbed through the intestinal wall directly into the bloodstream. Effects kick in 10 to 15 minutes after insertion and last up to 8 hours.

Another form of application is through the skin using transdermal patches and topicals. Transdermal patches take effect in 10 to 15 minutes and can last 8 to 12 hours. They deliver the chemicals straight to the bloodstream. Transdermal patches and suppositories are ideal for people who have severe nausea or who are unable to ingest or inhale.

Topicals are cannabis-infused balms, oils, and lotions that absorb through the skin and activate the CB2 receptors. They provide localized treatment without the psychoactive effects. Unlike transdermal patches and suppositories, topicals are nonpsychoactive because they can't get into the bloodstream. Topicals provide localized relief of pain, sore muscles, tension, and inflammation. They may also relieve psoriasis, dermatitis, itching, headaches, and cramping.

Everyone processes cannabis differently, so be aware that what works for one person might not work for you. Cannabis might make one person experience stress relief and sedation while it makes another feel overstimulated and energized. Several factors can contribute to these differences:

- strain used
- amount consumed
- method of consumption (inhaled, ingested, transdermal)
- environment or setting
- mind-set or mood
- recent experience or history with cannabis use
- nutrition or diet
- stomach contents
- metabolism, hormones, and biochemistry
- drugs, medicine, and supplements used

The endocannabinoid system is a relatively new discovery and isn't fully understood, and there may be unknown interactions that can be dangerous to cannabis users. For example, people with preexisting psychiatric disorders, such as schizophrenia, or a family history of mental illness may have negative reactions to marijuana. It can lead to a very negative experience (panic, anxiety, or paranoia) or an acute psychotic state. Some researchers believe there is a link between marijuana use and the precipitation of schizophrenia.[92] If you do have a family history of psychosis, particularly schizophrenia, consider the potential risks before trying cannabis yourself.

Anyone who is on a transplant list should speak with a doctor about cannabis use and candidacy for a transplant. Some transplant centers have a substance abuse policy that may reject cannabis users from their list of patients, despite recent findings that marijuana may help prevent transplant rejection.[93] Several organizations are fighting to ban the rejection of candidates using cannabis, but if you are on a transplant list, check with your doctor to make the best decision for you.

The elderly must be mindful that cannabis can cause dizziness or disturb balance coordination. A slip or fall could cause a host of other problems.

People with heart problems should consult a physician before using marijuana. Cannabis can cause the heart rate to increase. In rare

92. R. Radjakrishnan et al. "Gone to Pot—A Review of the Association between Cannabis and Psychosis," *Frontiers in Psychiatry* 5 (May 2014): 54. doi:10.3389/fpsyt.2014.00054. **93.** J. M. Sido et al., "Δ9-Tetrahydrocannabinol Attenuates Allogeneic Host-Versus-Graft Response and Delays Skin Graft Rejection Through Activation of Cannabinoid Receptor 1 and Induction of Myeloid-Derived Suppressor Cells," *Journal of Leukocyte Biology* 98, no. 3 (September 2015): 435–47. doi:10.1189/jlb.3A0115-030RR.

cases, it can double. There isn't enough research to conclusively say that cannabis is bad for people with heart problems, but some cardiologists and researchers warn against its use by patients with heart problems.

In a 2012 study, researchers found a link between cannabis and fertility issues in men.[94] Regular cannabis users had a lower sperm count than non-cannabis users.

Teens should steer clear of marijuana for now. There is conflicting evidence that children who use cannabis before age 16 may be susceptible to changes in the brain. More research is needed, but we advise keeping children and teens away from marijuana unless there is severe medical need.

Women who are pregnant, trying to get pregnant, or breastfeeding may also want to abstain from cannabis use. While there is no clear evidence that marijuana is harmful to mother or child, further studies are needed to be absolutely sure.

---

94. C. M. Fronczak, et al., "The Insults of Illicit Drug Use on Male Fertility," *Journal of Andrology* 33, no. 4 (July–August 2012): 515–28. doi:10.2164/jandrol.110.011874.

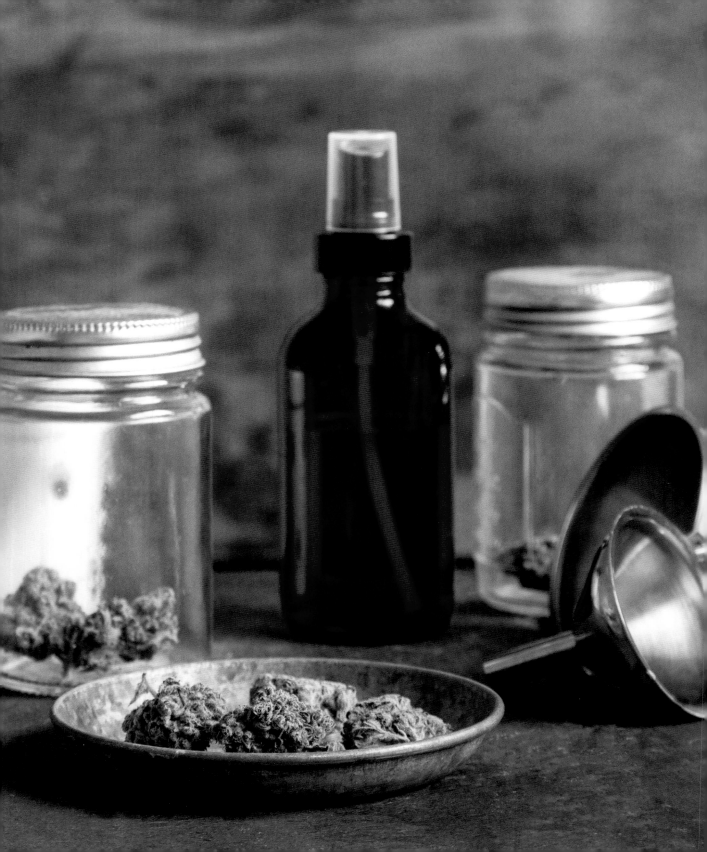

OBTAINING AND USING MARIJUANA

NOW THAT YOU understand the benefits and risks of using cannabis, it's time to go over the various methods of intake, as well as the logistics of obtaining, storing, and shopping for cannabis. It can be a simple choice or a complicated decision, depending upon your approach. Either way, there are certain considerations to be aware of when choosing a product and delivery method. After you review the delivery methods and products and decide on a course of treatment, it's important to keep a treatment log to help you understand what does and doesn't work for you.

DELIVERY METHODS

Smoking | Vaping | Dabbing | Tinctures Suppositories | Transdermal | Topicals Edibles | Capsules

There are a number of ways to use cannabis. Smoking a joint or lighting a pipe might be the delivery methods that come to mind, but vaporizing and dabbing are quickly picking up steam. There are also the beloved, yet controversial, edibles. Transdermal patches and suppositories have come on the scene in a big way; these methods are perhaps the most efficient way to absorb the medicine. Topicals are also a great option for people who need localized pain relief or want to avoid the psychotropic effects of marijuana. With all of these options, anyone can find their preferred method.

SMOKING

Smoking is the most common and recognizable delivery method. There are several possible methods of smoking, including joints, blunts, pipes, and bongs (water pipes). Smoking is prized for its convenience and simplicity, as well as the more natural and back-to-basics feel. However, the smoke, while not proven to inflict long-term harm, can be harsh on the lungs and throat.

Equipment Required

- Grinder
- Smoking apparatus (rolling paper, tobacco leaves, pipe, or bong)

Type of Marijuana Required

- Cannabis flower (buds)
- Optional concentrates such as kief, hash, oil, wax, budder, or live resin (see the "Medical Marijuana Products" chart on pages 61 and 62)

Associated Costs

- Cannabis flower (buds), typically $8 to $15 per gram
- Rolling papers, $1 to $5 per pack
- Pipe, $5 and up
- Bong, $30 and up

Who It's Best For

- Patients without lung or throat problems who are seeking rapid relief

HOW IT'S DONE

Both joints and blunts are smoked just like cigarettes. For a joint, cannabis is ground into crumbles before being rolled in a rolling paper of choice, such as paper made of rice, hemp, or cellulose. Blunts are similar, but tobacco leaves from cigar wrappers (which add flavor and nicotine) are used in place of the rolling paper. Concentrates can be added before rolling the joint or blunt, or the wrapped joint or blunt can be dipped in concentrated oil and/or rolled in kief (the plant resin).

Pipes and bongs eliminate the extra smoke from burning rolling papers or leaves. To smoke from one of these, place the cannabis loosely in the bowl. Cover the small hole in the air chamber near the bowl piece, called the *carb* or *carburetor*, if present, and light the cannabis. Draw in on the opening with your breath and release the carb just before finishing your inhale. Concentrates can be added on top of the cannabis in pipes and bongs for a potency boost.

Water pipes draw the smoke through a reservoir of water to cool the smoke before inhalation. Some people prefer this method, but be aware that studies have found that some of the THC/CBD is actually caught in the water although none of the harmful substances are. This means you will have to smoke more of the harmful chemicals to get the same amount of THC/CBD as you would without the presence of water.

It isn't advisable to smoke cannabis from a hookah (water pipes with long flexible tubes) because it burns the material faster than it can be smoked. It's also not recommended to smoke cannabis using cigarette filters, as they block a significant amount of THC, but not the harmful tars. Using filters would require smoking double the amount of tar to get the same amount of THC.

PROS AND CONS

Smoking cannabis introduces patients to, well, smoke. It can be harsh on the throat and lungs, and can increase the risk of bronchitis and other viral throat infections. When cannabis is smoked, a substantial amount of cannabinoids is lost. That being said, smoking requires no expensive equipment, the effects are felt quickly, and it is relatively easy to adjust your dose.

VAPING

Vaporizers heat cannabis to activate the cannabinoids and produce smokeless vapor. There are a few types of vaporizers to keep in mind, including large desktop vaporizers, small portable vaporizers, as well as conduction and convection vaporizers. Conduction heats the cannabis into smoke or vapor on a hot plate. Convection heats the air to activate the cannabis and release the cannabinoids/terpenes into the purest form through vapor without charring the material. Convection vaporizers give off the least amount of harmful chemicals and are the healthiest way to inhale cannabis.

Equipment Required
- Vaporizer (either desktop or portable)

Type of Marijuana Required
- Cannabis flower (buds) or concentrates such as oil, wax, budder, or live resin (see the "Medical Marijuana Products" chart on pages 61 and 62)

Associated Costs
- Ground cannabis or concentrate, $5 to $20 per gram depending on the market
- Desktop vaporizers, $150 to $600
- Portable vaporizers, $70 to $300

Who It's Best For
- Patients with or prone to throat or lung problems who want the easy, immediate relief of smoking without the harshness

HOW IT'S DONE

Vaporizers can be loaded with ground flower or concentrates. Portable vaporizers run by battery and desktop vaporizers must be plugged in to operate. Typically, they require some time to heat before inhaling the vapor. Refer to the manufacturer's instructions for how to operate and use a specific vaporizer.

PROS AND CONS

Vaping does not subject patients to the tar or harshness of smoke, nor does it result in the same level of terpene loss as smoking. Be aware that vaporizers, which also use water, can be prone to oxidization and rust, which is not a healthy substance to inhale. Moreover, if a vaporizer heats the cannabis above 365°F, it can release benzene, a common carcinogen found in tobacco. Some poorly made vaporizers have been found to contain chemical residue left over from the manufacturing process. Do your research before purchasing a vaporizer to ensure the quality meets your safety standards. Vaporizing is somewhat new, which means that the long-term effects of this method are unknown.

DABBING

Dabbing is the most controversial of all delivery methods. It involves heating a cannabis concentrate, such as shatter, on an extremely hot surface with a culinary torch before inhaling the smoke through a dab rig (a chambered glass pipe). This process has led to dabbing's unflattering depiction as the "crack" of the cannabis world.

Equipment Required
- Dab rig
- Culinary torch
- Dabber tool (a small rod used to scoop the extract)
- A nail with a titanium or quartz surface

Type of Marijuana Required
- Concentrates such as shatter, wax, budder, or live resin (see the "Medical Marijuana Products" chart on pages 61 and 62)

Associated Costs
- Concentrate, $30 to $50 per gram
- Dab rig, $20 to more than $1,000
- Dabber tools, $15 to $500
- Nail, $20 to $150
- Culinary torch, $15 to $50

Who It's Best For
- Patients dealing with severe pain or nausea who need immediate relief

HOW IT'S DONE
Dabbing should be done only by those who are knowledgeable with the process; if you are interested in this method, be sure to fully educate yourself on how it is done. Websites like The Cannabist and Leafly have sections on cannabis concentrates and how they're used. In general, when dabbing, heat up the nail with the culinary torch until it begins to glow, scoop the concentrate with the dabber tool, and start inhaling through the dab rig as you slide the concentrate from the dabber tool onto the heated nail. When the concentrate has melted and no more vapor is coming out, exhale.

PROS AND CONS
Dabbing provides high potency with immediate effects and minimal smoke. The high potency of dabbing can lead to very uncomfortable highs and, in some cases, passing out. To achieve the same level of effect that dabbing can provide, patients would have to smoke a large amount of cannabis or wait up to 3 hours with edibles.

TINCTURES

Cannabis tinctures are liquid extracts made with alcohol or vegetable glycerin. They are administered under the tongue. Because they require no equipment or preparation, they are convenient and easy to use.

Equipment Required

- None

Type of Marijuana Required

- Prepared tincture (see page 119 for a guide to making your own)

Associated Costs

- 1 ounce (about 600 drops), $30 to $80 depending on the product and market

Who It's Best For

- Patients who aren't willing or able to smoke or vape
- Patients who want a faster onset than edibles provide
- Elderly patients

HOW IT'S DONE

A few drops are administered under the tongue, where it enters the bloodstream more rapidly than edibles.

PROS AND CONS

There is no smoke or vapor, which is better for your lungs. It is also discreet; no smoke means no smell (aside from the smell of the tincture). Adjusting the level of the dose is relatively easy. Onset of effects begins quickly, within 5 to 15 minutes. Effects last about 30 minutes to 2 hours (not as long as edibles). The taste of tinctures can sometimes be unpleasant.

SUPPOSITORIES

A suppository is a small, bullet-shaped mass that is inserted into the rectum. Cannabis suppositories may be better absorbed by the body than taking cannabis by mouth. One study showed the absorption rate to be twice as effective as oral administration.[95] Suppositories are a good alternative for people who don't wish to smoke or ingest marijuana.

Equipment Required
- None

Type of Marijuana Required
- Suppository (see page 124 for a guide to making your own)

Associated Costs
- Suppository, $5 to $30 depending on the market

Who It's Best For
- Patients with an impaired oral route due to vomiting, throat injury, or extreme nausea
- Elderly patients who can't smoke or swallow pills
- Patients with rectal or pelvic disease, inflammatory bowel disease, or hemorrhoids

HOW IT'S DONE

Before inserting into the rectum, make sure the suppository is firm. If it's not firm, place it in the freezer until it reaches the desired consistency. Insert with clean hands or while wearing a medical glove. The suppository should ideally be placed around 1 to 1.5 inches (2.5 to 4 centimeters) into the rectum, just past the anal sphincter. Insert the suppository when you don't expect a bowel movement for at least an hour.

PROS AND CONS

Suppositories are thought to provide excellent absorption rates, superior to both inhalation and oral ingestion. Effects begin rapidly, within 10 to 15 minutes, and last for 4 to 8 hours. Insertion can be a little uncomfortable for some, and suppositories can leak during flatulence or a bowel movement. A suppository must be cool in temperature to be firm enough to insert.

---

95. Marilyn A. Huestis, "Human Cannabinoid Pharmacokinetics," *Chemistry & Biodiversity* 4, no. 8 (August 2007): 1770–804. doi:10.1002/cbdv.200790152.

TRANSDERMAL

Transdermal delivery is quite different from topicals. Instead of localized treatment, transdermal patches directly enter the bloodstream and provide treatment throughout the body. They also transmit the psychotropic effects of THC. Treatment is released slowly, peaking at 4 hours after application.

Equipment Required

- None

Type of Marijuana Required

- Transdermal patch

Associated Costs

- Transdermal patch, $18 to $30

Who It's Best For

- Patients with an impaired oral route due to vomiting, throat injury, or extreme nausea
- Elderly patients who can't smoke or swallow pills

HOW IT'S DONE

Using an alcohol wipe, wash a patch of skin with visible veins, such as the inside of your wrist. Apply the patch to the cleansed area. Refer to the manufacturer's instructions for complete details.

PROS AND CONS

Patches don't involve smoke, vapor, or smell. The patches last 8 to 12 hours, releasing small doses slowly. The transdermal delivery system is also believed to be very efficient, but no conclusive studies have been performed. Some people have had trouble properly adhering the patches to their skin, and others have found it hard to remove the plastic from the sticky part of the patch. Patches are only available to patients with access to well-stocked dispensaries. Overall, it seems to be a very promising delivery method.

TOPICALS

Cannabis topicals are infused lotions, oils, and salves that are rubbed on the skin for localized treatment and pain relief. Topicals don't enter the bloodstream; rather, they absorb into the skin and activate the CB2 receptors, providing nonpsychoactive treatment.

Equipment Required

- None

Type of Marijuana Required

- Topical treatment (see pages 125 to 127 for a guide to making your own)

Associated Costs

- Range of products (including lip balm, lotion, body balms, and body oil), $5 to $60

Who It's Best For

- Patients with arthritis, localized pain or inflammation, psoriasis, dermatitis, chronic itching, headaches, cramps, and lupus

HOW IT'S DONE

Rub the topical on the affected area.

PROS AND CONS

Topicals provide nonpsychoactive, localized pain relief and treatment. However, they don't help all conditions where activation of the CB1 receptors is required. Because new research is being conducted all the time, the list of applicable medical conditions will likely grow.

EDIBLES

This category includes any food or beverage that contains cannabis. Edibles are beloved by many for their simplicity, prolonged duration, and the fact that no smoking is involved. They have a somewhat controversial reputation for a couple of reasons. Because any food or drink can be made into a marijuana edible, there is a fear of accidental or purposeful "drugging" of unknowing consumers. Therefore, always label your edibles and keep them away from children and pets. Also, if you are unfamiliar with the dosing of a particular edible, it can be easy to overdo it.

Equipment Required

- None

Type of Marijuana Required

- Infused edible (see part 3 of this book, Recipes for Remedies and Edibles, for recipes)

Associated Costs

- Range of edibles, $10 to $50 per 100 mg of THC

Who It's Best For

- Patients who do not or cannot smoke or need a long-acting solution
- Patients with insomnia, Crohn's disease, irritable bowel syndrome (IBS), or gastro-intestinal issues

HOW IT'S DONE

Medically dosing with cannabis-infused edibles is pretty simple—you just eat them! Start with a small dose, about 2.5 to 5 mg of THC, and see how it affects you. Depending on your metabolism, it can take an hour or so for the effects to kick in. Peak effects usually occur at about 4 hours. Edibles are most effectively consumed in small morsels, ideally with a good amount of fat, on an empty stomach.

PROS AND CONS

The effects of ingesting cannabis have a slow onset but last longer than when cannabis is inhaled. Edibles provide a more psychoactive experience than inhalation. The dose can be difficult to predict, depending on the contents of your stomach at the time.

CAPSULES

Cannabis capsules, also known as canna-capsules, are food-grade capsules that have been filled with concentrated cannabis oil. These can be swallowed as you would an ordinary pill. Capsules provide similar effects as edibles, and are ideal for those who wish to ingest cannabis but don't desire the added calories.

Equipment Required

- None

Type of Marijuana Required

- Canna-capsules (see page 109 for instructions on how to make them)

Associated Costs

- Canna-capsules, around $5 per pill

Who It's Best For

- Patients who do not want to or cannot smoke
- Patients who are too nauseated to eat edibles or are on restricted diets

HOW IT'S DONE

Capsules should be taken with water and a little food, ideally with a good amount of fat, for the fastest and greatest effect.

PROS AND CONS

Capsules are a simple, smokeless way to ingest a standardized amount of cannabis. They have a slow onset (taking anywhere from 30 minutes to 3 hours to kick in) and a long duration (4 to 8 hours). Like edibles, they may provide a more psychoactive experience. Capsules provide a fairly consistent experience, although effects are influenced by the stomach contents.

BIOAVAILABILITY AND DOSING

Bioavailability is a measure of the absorption rates of a drug. For cannabis, it is a fraction or percentage of the inhaled or ingested cannabinoids present in the bloodstream. There are many factors that affect the bioavailability of the various delivery methods for cannabis, such as experience of the user, potency of the cannabis, method of delivery, stomach contents, metabolism, and biochemistry. However, there is still much we don't know, so further research is needed for a more complete picture.

One study found inhalation resulted in an absorption rate of 10 to 45 percent, with bioavailability peaking 3 to 10 minutes after inhalation.[96] Oral administration resulted in an absorption rate of 4 to 14 percent in one study[97] and 10 to 20 percent in another,[98] with peak bioavailability usually 1 to 2 hours after ingestion. Under-the-tongue absorption resulted in a 13 percent absorption while ingestion resulted in 5 percent. However, THC is converted in the liver into a metabolite 11-hydroxy-THC, which is considered twice as potent as THC and lasts twice as long. This metabolite isn't accounted for in the bioavailability of THC. Fatty foods have been found to increase absorption rates of ingested cannabis. Rectal administration was found to have a 13.5 percent absorption rate.[99]

Everyone reacts differently to the various delivery methods and strains. It's definitely worth taking the time to find the right product, dose, and delivery method for you. As stated earlier, when ingesting cannabis, start with low dosages of about 2.5 to 5 mg of THC, then wait at least 4 hours before having more. If inhaling, take a couple puffs and wait 15 minutes before increasing your dose.

Every time you medicate with cannabis, your reaction might be a bit different. The strain and strength of the cannabis, as well as anything you have recently eaten, might play into it. The only reliable way to achieve the same effects would be to have the same strain from the same grower's batch, or the same product, under the same conditions. With all the variables in life, this may be difficult to do. It's best to proceed with caution by trying a lower dose and waiting to experience the effects before deciding to have more.

It's important to keep a record of what works, what doesn't work, and why. Keep a log of your cannabis use to find the right dose and delivery method for you. At the end of this chapter, you'll find a treatment log you can use for this purpose.

96. F. Grotenhermen, "Pharmacokinetics and Pharmacodynamics of Cannabinoids," *Clinical Pharmacokinetics* 42, no. 4 (2003): 327–60, www.ncbi.nlm.nih.gov/pubmed/12648025. **97.** R. Brenneisen et al., "The Effect of Orally and Rectally Administered Delta 9-Tetrahydrocannabinol on Spasticity: A Pilot Study with 2 Patients," *International Journal of Clinical Pharmacology and Therapeutics* 34, no. 10 (October 1996): 446–52. **98.** B. R. Martin et al., "Chemistry and Pharmacology of Cannabis." In: H. Kalant, W. A. Corrigall, W. Hall, R. G. Smart, eds. "The Health Effects of Cannabis." Toronto: CAMH (1999): 19–68. **99.** R. Brenneisen et al., "The Effect of Orally and Rectally Administered Delta 9-Tetrahydrocannabinol on Spasticity: A Pilot Study with 2 Patients," *International Journal of Clinical Pharmacology and Therapeutics* 34, no. 10 (October 1996): 446–52.

WHAT TO DO IF YOU'VE HAD TOO MUCH

Too much cannabis can present some unpleasant side effects, including extreme anxiety, paranoia, hallucinations, dizziness, sweating, nausea, and vomiting. There has never been a lethal overdose reported, so if you do experience uncomfortable side effects, try to remember that you will be back to normal in several hours once it wears off.

Ask someone to watch over you during this time. In the unlikely case you develop symptoms such as trouble breathing, pale skin, fast heart rate, and/or unresponsiveness, they should call 911 or bring you to an emergency care center.

If you can, lie down and try to sleep it off. If not, there are a few things you can do to ease the effects. For example, if you have a CBD-dominant strain or concentrate on hand, inhale or ingest that if you can. As mentioned earlier, CBD has been found to inhibit the psychoactive effect of THC. Also, stay hydrated with non-caffeinated, nonalcoholic drinks, and be sure to eat something hearty if nausea and vomiting are not an issue.

Some people find relief by chewing a few black peppercorns or inhaling the scent of pine essential oil (both black pepper and pine contain terpenes found in cannabis). You can also try going for a walk to clear your head and get your blood pumping. Another approach is to distract yourself from the unpleasant effects by staying busy; you can watch a funny movie or TV show, draw/paint/color, listen to your favorite music, or play a lighthearted video game.

THOUGHTS AND EXPERIENCES

I have chronic pain in my neck and shoulders from a car accident I was in as a teenager. I had been to every kind of doctor, but I hadn't found any significant relief until marijuana. Cannabis has helped me get off pain medication and has been the best treatment for me.

Before I started using medicinal marijuana, there were times I couldn't get out of bed. I relied on hydrocodone to get me through the day. But the medicine made me sick, and I felt a dependency starting to develop. Acupuncture helped for a while, but the pain always came back and the treatment was too expensive to maintain.

I joined a support group for patients living with chronic pain, and that is where I learned about treating the pain with cannabis. Some people in the group reported that cannabis helped their pain and anxiety and recommended a doctor who could write a recommendation for a medical marijuana card.

When I got my card, I began experimenting with the different methods. I found that edibles provide the best relief for me. Now I have a cannabis caramel a couple times a day when my pain comes back. It is a low-dose edible with equal parts THC and CBD, so it doesn't make me too goofy. The pain is pretty much gone when the medication kicks in, enough for me to go about my day feeling normal. I live in a state with a medical marijuana program. If I didn't, I would probably move. —**L. Stevenson**, California

Strains— Do They Matter?

While strains, or genetic variants of cannabis, can guide your purchase, it's important to pay attention to the cannabinoid and terpene profiles to find the right cannabis for you. Cannabinoids and terpenes can vary significantly within the same strain from grower to grower. The strain may be mislabeled or the growing, curing, or storage conditions may be just different enough to cause variations. Medical research is not strain-specific, but it does look into cannabinoids for specific conditions. While all cannabis produces a set of similar effects, the cannabinoid and terpene content can yield markedly unique effects.

Terpenes are basically essential oils with very unique smells, but they do affect your overall cannabis experience. If the dispensary or seller doesn't have a cannabinoid or terpene profile, you can let your nose guide you. For a reference on terpene smell and effects, see page 42 in chapter 2. Smell every strain before you use it and lock that scent away in your memory. Your nose will remember that smell, and if it was a pleasant experience, seek it out. Jot the smell and taste down in your treatment log.

SHOPPING GUIDE

Trying medical marijuana for the first time can be exciting and a little nerve-racking, but there's no need to be overly concerned. If you follow your doctor's directions and listen to the advice of your budtender (the medical marijuana dispensary worker), you will likely have a very pleasant experience.

To begin your search for the right product, locate a dispensary. To find dispensaries close to you, visit weedmaps.com or leafly.com. These websites have menus of the shops' offerings. In some cases, the strains on their menus include the cannabinoid and terpenes profiles, which is great for doing research beforehand. They also post reviews from patients, which may be helpful. These sites are a great place to start your dispensary search, but nothing beats a face-to-face conversation with a dispensary's budtenders. Knowledgeable, caring staff can make all the difference. The workers at a good medicine-focused dispensary will ask about your treatment plan and goals. They will work with you to find the appropriate cannabis products. If you don't feel comfortable in a dispensary, don't hesitate to move on to the next one until you find the right match.

In your search for a strain of cannabis that offers the effects and treatment you need, there are certain things to watch out for and avoid. Ask the budtender about cannabis testing requirements and only purchase products that have tested negative for pesticides, contaminants, mold, and mildew. You don't want to inhale or ingest any of these harmful substances.

When you enter a dispensary, you may be taken aback by the selection. There are flower (buds), concentrates, edibles, topicals, and tinctures—and subcategories within these categories! Don't be afraid to ask questions until you understand the options, their uses, and effects. The following table provides a basic overview to get you started.

MEDICAL MARIJUANA PRODUCTS

Description	Required Equipment	Pros	Cons
FLOWER (BUDS) The flowers, or buds, of the cannabis plant are divided by strains and generally sorted into three categories: *indica*, *sativa*, and hybrid.	Flower can be smoked, vaped, or turned into concentrates or extractions. A pipe, bong, vaporizer, or rolling paper is needed for inhalation.	Flower is the most natural way to consume cannabis. There is no risk of inhaling solvents.	Flower can be harsh on the lungs and throat when smoked. It is the lowest-potency product.
WAX Wax is waxy or crumbly bits of concentrate.	Wax can be inhaled with a vaporizer, pipe, or dab rig.	Wax has a high potency.	Wax is a processed product. Long-term effects are unknown. Smoking anything can be harsh on the lungs and throat.
BUDDER Budder is whipped wax/oil with a dough-like texture.	It can be inhaled with a vaporizer, pipe, or dab rig.	Budder has a high potency.	Budder is a processed product. Long-term effects are unknown. Smoking anything can be harsh on the lungs and throat.
KIEF Kief is powdery flakes from the plant resin.	It can be inhaled with a vaporizer, on top of flower in a pipe, or in a joint with flower.	Kief has a natural, high potency.	Smoking anything can be harsh on the lungs and throat.
HASH Hash is a soft, pliant, paste-like concentrate made from kief. It will become less pliant over time with exposure to oxygen.	It can be smoked in a hash pipe, mixed into joints, or inhaled with a vaporizer.	Hash has a high potency.	Hash is a processed product. Smoking anything can be harsh on the lungs and throat.
TINCTURE Tincture is an alcohol- or glycerin-based extract taken orally.	It's taken under the tongue with no equipment needed.	Tincture has a high potency and is smokeless.	A tincture is a processed product. It can have an unpleasant taste.

▶

Description	Required Equipment	Pros	Cons
OIL			
This is a dark, gooey, concentrated oil typically found in plastic syringes. It's made from solvents such as butane, ethanol, CO_2, isopropyl, alcohol, or hexane.	Oil can be smoked in a pipe or vaporizer, mixed in with buds in a joint, taken under the tongue like a tincture, inserted into pill capsules, or added to food.	Oil has a high potency.	This is a processed product. Long-term effects are unknown. There's a risk of remaining solvents or harmful chemicals in concentrated oil.
LIVE RESIN			
It's created with fresh, live plants that have not yet been dried, optimizing the amount of natural terpenes.	Live resin can be inhaled with a vaporizer or dab rig.	Live resin has a high potency and preserved terpenes.	This is a processed product. Long-term effects are unknown. Smoking anything can be harsh on the lungs and throat.
SHATTER			
Shatter is a semitransparent sheet of glass-like concentrate.	Shatter is often inhaled with a dab rig, although it can be inhaled with a vaporizer if you are able to break off a small, pliable piece.	Shatter has a high potency.	This is a processed product. Long-term effects are unknown. Smoking anything can be harsh on the lungs and throat.

TIPS FOR PATIENTS ON A BUDGET

Grow your own, if permitted in your state. There are many helpful resources online to get you started. You can start with a seed, or better yet, a clone (an immature baby plant) from your local dispensary or a grower friend. You can also read *The Cannabis Grow Bible* by Greg Green for a comprehensive growing guide.

Save the used flower from your vaporizer. Referred to as ABV (already been vaped), this can replace or be added to the flower you use to make edibles.

Buy in bulk up to the amount permitted in your state. Dispensaries usually offer a discount for large purchases.

Tell your budtender. If you are on a budget, let your budtender know. They can help find the most cost-effective products and deals.

Look for deals. Research dispensaries on leafly.com or weedmaps.com and look for daily deals, such as Free Joint Fridays or

Medible Mondays. By hitting dispensaries for the products you need on certain days, you can save a lot of money. You can also find deals for first-time patients.

Follow the free stuff. Subscribe to all your local marijuana publications and keep an eye out for cannabis-related events. There are often vendors at these events giving out free products.

Don't waste. Stop inhaling or ingesting once you've had enough. When you reach the dosage level that achieves the treatment or relief you need, stop. Don't overdo it, and don't waste valuable medicine.

Store your cannabis properly. If stored in poor conditions, the plant will degrade and become less potent.

Share, trade, and barter. Create a network of friends who also medicate with cannabis, and create a sharing economy. If you make topicals, trade some for free flower or shake. Maybe you give them flower and they turn it into concentrate. There are a lot of talented patients out there who love to share, trade, and offer advice.

Your First Trip to the Dispensary

Your first visit to a dispensary is likely to be an exciting and memorable experience. Bring a photo ID and your medical marijuana card every time you visit a dispensary. Dispensaries are generally a cash-only business and have a lot of security, so you may have to provide ID each time you enter.

Tell the staff you're a new patient and this is your first time in a dispensary. They will give you paperwork to sign and check you in before setting you up with a budtender to walk you through your options. Be courteous to the staff and other customers and follow the dispensary's rules.

Tell your budtender that you're a new patient. Explain the treatment you are seeking. Ask if they have any advice, and inquire about deals and services offered, like e-mail newsletters with special offers and news, delivery services, or offerings like Free Joint Fridays.

There are a lot of options for cannabis products. It may help to peruse the shop's menu online before visiting so you're not overwhelmed and can prepare questions for the budtenders. Don't touch the cannabis flower until given permission—this is bad etiquette. Not only could you contaminate it with your germs, but you could also decrease the potency by disturbing the trichomes.

Purchase cannabis in small amounts until you know what works for you. Your purchased products will come in childproof containers and opaque "exit bags." Depending on your state laws, you may need to put the purchased products in your car's trunk for transporting home.

If you have a negative experience, let the manager know and write a review of your experience on leafly.com or weedmaps.com. Don't let a bad experience ruin medical cannabis for you. Try another shop as if it were your first time. Your first visit is likely to be a great experience, so just relax and enjoy the ride!

MEDICAL MARIJUANA TREATMENT LOG

To discover what works best for you, keep a detailed log of all cannabis use, including the delivery method, product used, dose, and the effects. Keep this log as long as it takes to find a regimen that works for you. Record the date, the symptoms you want to combat, how much discomfort you are in before using medical marijuana, the delivery method, the cannabis product, the dose, the cannabinoid and terpene profile of the product if available, description of the effects, your discomfort level after using medical marijuana, and whether you would use the product again. Try to be consistent and thorough when keeping a log. This will be an important key to finding out your optimal treatment.

A sample log has been provided on the next page. Feel free to modify the log by adding additional spaces to record your experiences with doctors, dispensaries, delivery services, and budtenders, too.

LOGISTICS

Storing Cannabis

Cannabis is a hardy plant and, when stored properly, can keep for a couple years. If you are going to purchase an amount of cannabis that will last you longer than a week, there are some important things to keep in mind to maintain freshness and potency.

When handling cannabis, be gentle and avoid touching it too much. The crystal-like trichomes can fall off and the cannabis will lose potency. Trichomes, as you've learned, are the resinous compounds on the plant, and home to all the important cannabinoids and terpenes. The cannabis you buy will have been carefully dried and cured, and the storing process is extremely important.

Separate strains into different containers to maintain their unique flavor profiles. Marijuana is best stored in a cool, dark place in an airtight container with a neutral charge (like glass). If the container can be vacuum sealed, even better. Oxygen exposure can degrade some cannabinoids. High temperatures and sunlight can also degrade the THC into a less-desirable CBN (a cannabinoid known for extreme sedation). Keep it out of the refrigerator, which has a relatively high humidity. High humidity can cause mold and mildew growth, which is very unhealthy if inhaled or ingested. You want to maintain a humidity ideally between 50 to 65 percent relative humidity (RH). Humidity lower than 50 percent, as well as freezing temperatures, can dry out the trichomes, creating harsh smoke and loss of potency.

Do not use tobacco humidors, as they contain natural essential oils in the cedar that can alter and affect the flavor profile of the cannabis. Although some say that plastic bags work well, it seems that static electricity attracts the resin and some potency may be lost. Another reason to avoid plastic bags is that some contain dioxin, a chemical

MEDICAL MARIJUANA TREATMENT LOG

Keeping a detailed log of your cannabis use can help you figure out the best regimen for your needs. Record the date, the symptoms you want to combat, how much discomfort you are in before using medical marijuana, the delivery method (joint, tincture, edible, etc.), the product (strain name, product name), the dose (grams for flower or concentrate, milligrams of THC, number of pills, number of tincture drops, etc.), the cannabinoid and terpene profile of the product if available, description of the effects (time to onset, how you were affected, duration of effects), your discomfort level after using medical marijuana (did the cannabis relieve your pain or did it cause pain/discomfort?), and whether you would use the product again.

Date	My Symptoms and Health Needs		Pre-Medicated Discomfort Level (on a scale from 1 to 10)
Delivery Method	Product	Dose	Cannabinoids and Terpenes
Description of Effects		Post-Medicated Discomfort Level (on a scale from 1 to 10)	Use Again? Why/Why not?
Notes			

compound considered to be an environmental pollutant. If glass jars are not an option, your best bet is to keep your cannabis in brown paper bags. Gently squeeze the air out and place the paper bag inside a sealable plastic bag. There are also several products on the market for properly storing cannabis. Boveda, Cannador, and The Bureau offer consumer solutions for storing your cannabis in ideal conditions.

Storing Concentrates and Edibles

When storing your concentrates and edibles, follow instructions from the manufacturer, if available. In general, store edibles as you would everyday perishable foods. Baked goods can be frozen for long-term storage without harming the potency. Hard candies, caramels, and chocolate can be kept at room temperature.

Store canna-butter (see our recipe for canna-butter on page 106) the same way you would store regular butter. Keep what you will use for a week or so in the refrigerator. Wrap it well and label it with the date, strain, and potency. If you don't know the potency, just note whether it is mild, medium, or strong, or at least how much is the right dose for you. If you plan to keep canna-butter longer than a week or so, it's best to store it in the freezer.

Store tinctures in a cool, dark place in an airtight glass container. Concentrates are perishable; the oils from the plant can turn rancid. Some choose to keep their cannabis oils in the refrigerator to keep them at a controlled temperature. However, it's fine to store the oil at room temperature—just keep it out of the sunlight or heat. Refrigerating cannabis oils and waxes can prolong their life. Avoid refreezing any of the concentrates.

Equipment Care

Always clean residue from your equipment. You can buy cleaners at glass shops or use a solution of salt and alcohol and let it sit for about an hour before rinsing thoroughly. The resin is very sticky, so you might want to use a cotton swab or pipe cleaner to help with the tough spots. Keep clean glass pieces on a shelf or in a padded box.

Troubleshooting FAQ

The following covers a number of frequently asked questions about marijuana use and potential issues or concerns. Hopefully, these will address some questions you might still have regarding logistics.

How can I get rid of weed smell?

There are a number of ways to get rid of the smell of marijuana. You can use an air-neutralizing product, open windows to get cross ventilation, or light an aromatic candle. Some people cook something with a strong smell, such as a garlicky tomato sauce, to cover the aroma. You can buy products to blow your smoke to neutralize the smell, such as the Smokebuddy personal air filter. You can also make a sploof, a homemade filter for blowing smoke through, with an empty toilet paper or paper towel roll, dryer sheets, and a clean sock. To make this gadget, stuff several dryer sheets into the empty roll and cover one end of the roll with a sock. Blow the smoke or vapor through the open end of the roll to counteract the smell of the smoke and odor.

Will marijuana use give me a hangover?

It's rare to experience a marijuana hangover. It can happen, but generally only if you have really overdone it, particularly with edibles. Because it takes longer to metabolize an edible, the effects may still be present in the morning. The effects will not be nearly as bad as an alcohol hangover; you may feel a little groggy and your motor coordination and reaction time may be a bit slower than normal. Take a hot shower or bath, eat a full meal, drink plenty of water, and have a cup of coffee or tea. If you still feel the hangover, take a walk or a nap and be patient.

Should I stop taking my other medicine if I am switching to cannabis?

Do not stop taking any prescription medicine without talking with your doctor.

If my friend is interested in trying my marijuana, can I share it or sell it?

If you live in a state where marijuana is recreationally legal, you can *share* it with your friends, as long as they are 21 or over and in good emotional health. It is illegal to sell cannabis without a license. Penalties for breaking the law can be harsh, so be sure to act responsibly.

THOUGHTS AND EXPERIENCES

Patients have been asking me to write them a script for cannabis for more than 12 years. Until recently, it wasn't possible; it wasn't even something I would have considered. I had tried smoking in college, and I wasn't impressed. However, over the last year, I have seen some changes in my practice. Three of my patients have been using cannabis for various reasons. The first has a seizure disorder, the second has a back injury, and the third has severe bipolar disorder.

The patient with the seizures is markedly better. Her daily seizures have reduced to maybe one or two a month. The patient with the back injury has stopped taking pain pills. While my bipolar patient still has ups and downs, she reports that her downs are less severe and that she is not nearly as manic.

A few months ago, I began using cannabis myself instead of sleeping pills to treat my insomnia, and I have had great success. I continue to be impressed by the medicinal benefits of the drug, and I am looking forward to a broader adoption in the medical community. —**H. J.**, Colorado

If I need to drive my car, can I still use my marijuana product?

No. Driving while under the influence of marijuana is risky and illegal. Never drive (or operate heavy machinery) while experiencing cannabis's effects. If you need to go somewhere, call a taxi or ask a friend to drive you. Never smoke in a car, and if you are carrying cannabis, it is best to keep it in the trunk. None of the passengers in your vehicle should be using cannabis either.

Can I lose my job for using marijuana?

Yes, your employer has the right to fire you if you are found to be using medical marijuana even when you are off the job. Read through your company's HR policy to know your rights, as well as your company's rights. If you are a medical marijuana user and you are being drug tested at your place of employment, talk with your HR representative or a trusted supervisor and let them know your situation. Show them a note from your physician and tell them about how your use of cannabis has helped you. If you are using cannabis responsibly for a medical situation, we hope your employer sees it that way.

Can I smoke marijuana in public places like restaurants and bars?

No, marijuana cannot be used in a public place. Having a medical marijuana card or living in a state where recreational use is legal does not mean it can be used anywhere.

What is the minimum age for using marijuana?

You must be 21 or over to use marijuana in states where marijuana is legal unless you have a medical marijuana card.

If I'm traveling to another state, can I bring my marijuana with me?

No, you may not bring your cannabis across state lines since cannabis is still federally illegal.

What should I do if my marijuana has gone bad?

Cannabis can degrade and lose potency if exposed to sunlight, humidity, or extreme temperatures. But, if stored correctly, it will last a very long time. (See page 64 for tips on storing cannabis properly.) If you suspect your marijuana has developed mold or mildew, or looks or smells strange, discard it.

Where can I learn to grow marijuana?

Growing marijuana is relatively easy—there is a reason it is sometimes called weed. Refer to online guides or *The Cannabis Grow Bible* by Greg Green for full instructions on how to grow cannabis at home.

What should I do if I'm arrested for possession of cannabis?

Remember that there are still laws in effect that limit or prohibit the use of cannabis. If you are arrested, do not give the police permission to search your property and do not answer any questions. Be polite and courteous, but inform the officer that you are using your right to remain silent. Ask for an attorney. Police are allowed to use deception to get a confession, so, unfortunately, you may not be able trust what they tell or promise you. Remain silent until you consult with an attorney.

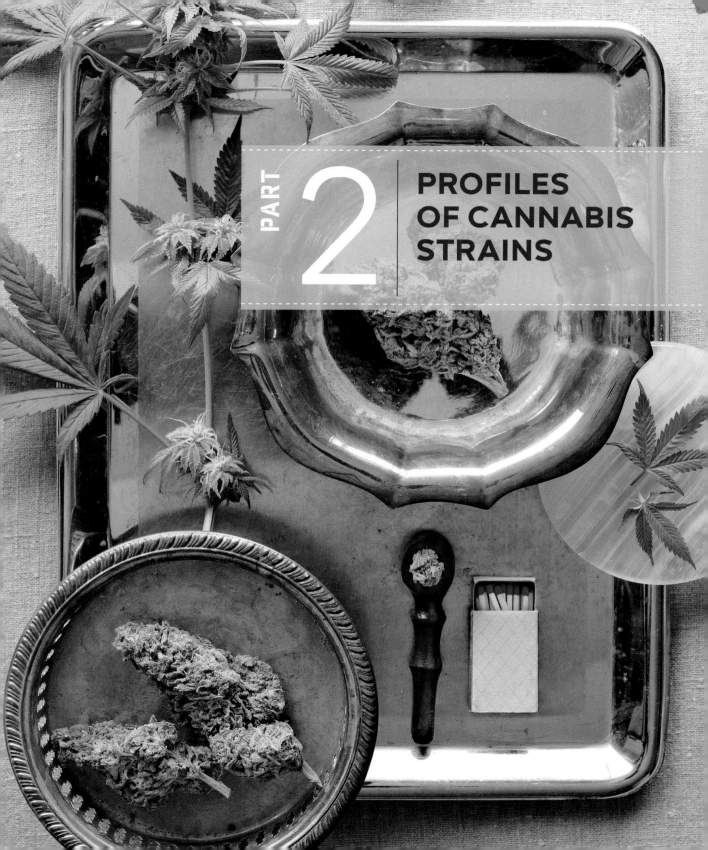

PART 2 | PROFILES OF CANNABIS STRAINS

Indicas are well loved because they are believed to offer a relaxing body high and to treat pain, spasms, anxiety, nausea, and insomnia. But as mentioned in chapter 1, this is not always the case, since researchers continue to find little difference in the observable effects between *indicas* and *sativas*. When selecting a strain, pay more attention to the available cannabinoid and terpene content of each strain to find the best fit for your symptoms.

INDICA STRAINS

THIS CHAPTER INCLUDES information on *indica* strains, including cannabinoid content, taste and aroma, potency effects (both medicinal and recreational), common medicinal uses, and potential unwanted effects (such as dizziness, dry eyes, and dry mouth). We include the percentage of THC and CBD content for each strain, and when possible, the percentages of other cannabinoids as well. These are average percentages, subject to change based on environmental variations. Just because the percentage of a certain cannabinoid isn't listed, that doesn't mean it's not present in the strain. Unfortunately, cannabinoids other than THC and CBD are still not as well known or tested and therefore are not as available for reporting.

It is also important to understand not only the differences among various strains, but also the potential differences between one strain from two different plants. Environmental factors such as temperature, sunlight, soil type, and nutrients can affect the final output and effects of a plant. While each strain has pretty defined genetics, don't be surprised if Bubba Kush from one grower isn't quite the same as Bubba Kush from another.

As you flip through this chapter, you will notice some pretty strange strain names. Sometimes, strains are named for their appearance, origin, or effects. Other times, they go by more creative names for marketing purposes or were created by recreational users from years ago just for the fun of it.

AFGHANI KUSH

One of the oldest strains, Afghani Kush's origins can be traced back to the mountains between the Afghanistan and Pakistan border. This relaxing, euphoric strain has great pain-relieving properties. Its high resin yield produces powerful sedating effects, making it excellent for nighttime use.

CANNABINOIDS
THC: 13.19 percent
CBD: 0.15 percent

POTENCY EFFECTS
Appetite-stimulating, euphoric, relaxing, sleep-inducing

Genetic History
Landrace Afghani Cultivar

Aroma and Taste
Sweet, orange, mango, earthy, woody

Conditions Treated
Arthritis, depression, insomnia, lack of appetite, migraines, nausea, pain relief, stress

Unwanted Effects
Dizziness, dry eyes, dry mouth, paranoia

BLUEBERRY

Blueberry produces euphoria and deep relaxation, making it excellent for nighttime use. This legendary strain won the 2000 *High Times* Cannabis Cup for Best *Indica*. It is loved for its pain- and stress-relieving properties, as well as its relaxing euphoria and sweet berry taste.

CANNABINOIDS
THC: 21 percent
CBD: 0.15 percent

POTENCY EFFECTS
Creative, euphoric, social, upbeat

Genetic History
Purple Thai, Highland Thai, Afghan *Indica*

Aroma and Taste
Blueberry, fruity, sweet

Conditions Treated
Anxiety, arthritis, headaches, migraines, PTSD, pain, sleep disorders, stress

Unwanted Effects
Dry eyes, dry mouth

BUBBA KUSH

This is a heavy-hitting *indica* with tranquilizing, muscle-relaxing effects. The original *indica* from which this strain was developed is commonly referred to as Pre 98 Bubba Kush or Straight Bubba. Many breeders have developed their own renditions of Bubba Kush, each slightly different but all with a powerful, sedating body high.

CANNABINOIDS
THC: 19.77 percent
CBD: 0.17 percent

POTENCY EFFECTS
Appetite-stimulating, contemplative, euphoric, narcotic, relaxing, sedating

----

Genetic History
Unknown, possibly O.G. Kush, West Coast Dog, Hindu Kush

Aroma and Taste
Coffee, earthy, sweet, spicy, piney, citrusy, bitter

Conditions Treated
Anorexia, migraines, multiple sclerosis, nausea, pain relief, sleep disorders

Unwanted Effects
Dizziness, dry eyes, dry mouth

CRITICAL KUSH

Critical Kush is an *indica* with a high THC count and a moderate level of CBD. It has a powerful, relaxing high that is perfect for nighttime treatment of pain, muscle spasms, and insomnia.

CANNABINOIDS
THC: 25 percent
CBD: 2.1 percent

POTENCY EFFECTS
Creative, focused, happy, uplifting

Genetic History
Critical Mass and O.G. Kush

Aroma and Taste
Woody, pungent, earthy

Conditions Treated
Muscle spasms, pain relief, sleep disorders, stress

Unwanted Effects
Dizziness, dry eyes, dry mouth

G-13

This *indica* provides a strong body high with an uplifting, joyful state of mind. The urban legend is that this strain was developed by the United States Central Intelligence Agency (CIA) from the best strains in the world at a secret location in Mississippi in the late 1960s. Regardless of the level of truth in this story, this strain offers a potent body high with negligible fatigue.

- -

CANNABINOIDS
THC: 19.45 percent
CBD: 0.17 percent

POTENCY EFFECTS
Cerebral, creative, euphoric, focusing, relaxing

- -

Genetic History
Unknown, rumored to be bred by the US government

Aroma and Taste
Minty, musky, spicy, sweet

Conditions Treated
Anorexia, anxiety disorder, arthritis, depression, lack of appetite, migraines, nausea, sleep disorders, stress

Unwanted Effects
Dry mouth, dry eyes

GRANDDADDY PURPLE

With its deep purple flowers and white resinous tips, this strain is quite attractive. It is a great choice for pain relief and is best taken at night. It will help you float away to sleep in a dreamy buzz.

- -

CANNABINOIDS
THC: 22.92 percent
CBD: 0.13 percent

POTENCY EFFECTS
Euphoric, relaxing, sedating

- -

Genetic History
Big Bud, Purple Urkle

Aroma and Taste
Berry, grape, sweet

Conditions Treated
Alzheimer's disease, headache, lack of appetite, migraines, nausea, pain relief, Parkinson's disease, sleep disorder

Unwanted Effects
Dizziness, dry eyes, dry mouth, paranoia

HASH PLANT

This resin-drenched strain offers a powerful body high with heavy narcotic effects. It took first place at Cannabis Cultures Toker's Bowl in 2004 and second place at the Highlife (Cup) Hemp Fair in 2002.

CANNABINOIDS
THC: 20.42 percent
CBD: 0.17 percent

POTENCY EFFECTS
Calming, narcotic, relaxing, sleep-inducing

Genetic History
Afghani Landrace, Northern Lights #1

Aroma and Taste
Earthy, spicy, sweet, woody

Conditions Treated
Appetite stimulant, depression, headache, nausea, pain relief, PMS, sleep disorders, stress

Unwanted Effects
Dry eyes, dry mouth, lethargy

HINDU KUSH

Also known as Afghanica, this pure *indica* strain originated in the Afghanistan and Pakistan region. It has a thick coat of trichomes, bringing calm and pain relief with a mid-level potency.

CANNABINOIDS
THC: 17.04 percent
CBD: 0.12 percent

POTENCY EFFECTS
Calming, euphoric, narcotic, sedating, sleep-inducing, relaxing, uplifting

----

Genetic History
Cultivated *Indica* Landrace

Aroma and Taste
Earthy, lemony, sweet, woody

Conditions Treated
Anorexia, anxiety, arthritis, depression, headache, nausea, pain relief, PTSD, sleep disorders, stress

Unwanted Effects
Dizziness, dry eyes, dry mouth, paranoia

KOSHER KUSH

This heavy-hitting *indica* strain is an excellent prescription for a good night's sleep. Despite its name, this strain is not actually kosher (to be kosher, it must meet certain guidelines and be blessed by a rabbi). It was, however, blessed with the *High Times* Cannabis Cup in 2015 for Best *Indica* Flower.

CANNABINOIDS
THC: 29.60 percent
CBD: 0.70 percent

POTENCY EFFECTS
Calming, euphoric,
narcotic, relaxing

Genetic History
Unknown

Aroma and Taste
Earthy, piney, woody

Conditions Treated
Anxiety disorder, insomnia,
pain relief, sleep apnea

Unwanted Effects
Dizziness, dry eyes, dry mouth

LA CONFIDENTIAL

This attractive strain is light green with frosted resinous tips and small purple leaves. It is a well-rounded strain that calms the body and mind, sending you into a pleasant slumber.

CANNABINOIDS
THC: 19 percent
THCV: 0.02 percent
CBD: 0.08 percent
CBG: 0.3 percent
CBL: 0.02 percent
CBN: 0.01 percent

POTENCY EFFECTS
Euphoric, happy, relaxing, sleep-
inducing, uplifting

Genetic History
O.G. LA Affie, Afghani

Aroma and Taste
Earthy, piney, pungent

Conditions Treated
Depression, insomnia,
lack of appetite, pain, stress

Unwanted Effects
Dizziness, dry eyes, dry mouth

MAPLE LEAF

This strain enhances creativity and focus, then progresses to sleepiness and fatigue. It's a great strain for meditation and sleep. This strain hails from Afghanistan, extracted before the Soviet invasion in 1979.

- -

CANNABINOIDS
THC: 17.49 percent
CBD: 0.14 percent

POTENCY EFFECTS
Calming, creative, narcotic, relaxing, sedating
- -

Genetic History
Afghani Landrace Strain

Aroma and Taste
Peppery, spicy, sweet

Conditions Treated
Anorexia, anxiety disorder, arthritis, depression, lack of appetite, migraines, nausea, sleep disorders, stress

Unwanted Effects
Dizziness, dry eyes, dry mouth, headache, lethargy, paranoia

MAZAR I SHARIF

This strain has a hard and fast body high; it's great for relieving chronic pain and getting a good night's sleep. This *indica* comes from the desert in northern Afghanistan, close to the border of Turkmenistan.

- -

CANNABINOIDS
THC: 15.96 percent
CBD: 0.16 percent

POTENCY EFFECTS
Euphoric, relaxing, sedating, sleep-inducing
- -

Genetic History
Landrace *Indica* Cultivar from northern Afghanistan

Aroma and Taste
Spicy, sweet, earthy, woody

Conditions Treated
Anxiety disorder, depression, pain relief, PMS, PTSD, sleep disorders, stress

Unwanted Effects
Dry eyes, dry mouth, paranoia

NORTHERN LIGHTS

This well-known *indica* strain is the parent of many award-winning strains, and a popular, beloved *indica* in its own right. It originated in Seattle in the late 1970s. It produces a powerful body high and a relaxing sense of euphoria.

CANNABINOIDS
THC: 16.53 percent
CBD: 0.15 percent

POTENCY EFFECTS
Calming, sleep-inducing, uplifting

Genetic History
Afghani *Indica* Cultivar

Aroma and Taste
Earthy, lemony, piney, spicy, sweet

Conditions Treated
Anxiety disorder, arthritis, cachexia, depression, migraines, nausea, pain relief, stress

Unwanted Effects
Anxiety, dizziness, dry eyes, dry mouth, paranoia

PURPLE KUSH

Sometimes called Oaksterdam based on its origins in Oakland, California, Purple Kush offers soothing pain relief and an easygoing high without being overly sedating. This *indica* is effective for treating pain, depression, and muscle spasms.

CANNABINOIDS
THC: 19.97 percent
CBD: 0.14 percent

POTENCY EFFECTS
Calming, blissful, relaxing, sedating

Genetic History
Hindu Kush, Purple Afghani

Aroma and Taste
Earthy, grape, piney, sweet

Conditions Treated
Anxiety disorder, depression, inflammation, muscle tension, pain relief, stress

Unwanted Effects
Dry mouth, lethargy

PURPLE URKLE

Also known as Purple Urple or The Urkle, this heavy-hitting *indica* hails from Northern California and offers full-body pain relief. It is ideal for nighttime use.

CANNABINOIDS
THC: 15.87 percent
CBD: 0.36 percent
CBN: 0.10 percent

POTENCY EFFECTS
Appetite-stimulating, euphoric, happy, sleep-inducing, relaxing

----

Genetic History
Mendocino Purps

Aroma and Taste
Sweet, berry, grape

Conditions Treated
Depression, insomnia, pain, stress

Unwanted Effects
Dizziness, dry eyes, dry mouth

SENSI STAR

Winner of 14 awards between 1999 and 2010, Sensi Star is among the most award-winning strains currently available. This *indica* packs a punch and is often recommended for patients with a high tolerance.

CANNABINOIDS
THC: 16.46 percent
CBD: 0.07 percent

POTENCY EFFECTS
Cerebral, contemplative, euphoric, uplifting

Genetic History
Afghani *Indica*, unknown

Aroma and Taste
Earthy, lemony, minty, piney, spicy

Conditions Treated
Anorexia, anxiety disorder, depression, glaucoma, headache, migraines, pain relief, PTSD, stress

Unwanted Effects
Dizziness, dry eyes, dry mouth, headache, lethargy

Sativas are preferred by those who believe they offer an uplifting, energetic experience without the sedating nature of *indicas*. But, as we reminded you in chapter 4, researchers continue to find little difference in the observable effects of *indicas* and *sativas*, so it is best to pay more attention to the available cannabinoid and terpene content when selecting a strain that best fits your needs.

SATIVA STRAINS

THIS CHAPTER INCLUDES information on cannabinoid content, taste and aroma, potency effects (both medicinal and recreational), common medicinal uses, and potential unwanted effects (such as dizziness, dry eyes, and dry mouth) of specific *sativa* strains. We include the percentage of THC and CBD content for each strain, and when possible, the percentages of other cannabinoids as well. These are average percentages, subject to change based on environmental variations. Just because the percentage of a certain cannabinoid isn't listed, that doesn't mean it's not present in the strain. Unfortunately, cannabinoids other than THC and CBD are still not as well known or tested and therefore are not as available for reporting.

It is also important to understand not only the differences among various strains, but also the potential differences between one strain from two different plants. Environmental factors such as temperature, sunlight, soil type, and nutrients can affect the final output and effects of a plant. While each strain has pretty defined genetics, don't be surprised if Cinex from one grower isn't quite the same as Cinex from another.

Just as in the last chapter, you will notice some bizarre (and even obscene) strain names. The names of strains can originate from their appearance, origin, or sometimes even a silly reference created years ago.

ACAPULCO GOLD

A high-quality *sativa* with a signature gold hue, Acapulco Gold is one of the best-known strains. It originated in, you guessed it, Acapulco.

CANNABINOIDS
THC: 23 percent
CBD: 0.70 percent

POTENCY EFFECTS
Energizing, euphoric, happy, relaxing, uplifting

Genetic History
Central American origins

Aroma and Taste
Earthy, woody, pungent

Conditions Treated
Depression, fatigue, lack of appetite, pain, PTSD, stress

Unwanted Effects
Dizziness, dry eyes, dry mouth, paranoia

ALASKAN THUNDERFUCK

Probably the strangest strain name (we didn't come up with these!), this strong *sativa* is also known as Matanuska Tundra by a few. It provides a relaxing, happy, euphoric high. It's ideal for morning or daytime use.

CANNABINOIDS
THC: 26 percent
CBD: 0.11 percent

POTENCY EFFECTS
Cerebral, happy, euphoric, energizing, relaxing, sedating, social, uplifting

----

Genetic History
North American *Sativa*, Russian *Ruderalis*, Afghani *Indica*

Aroma and Taste
Sweet, earthy, pungent

Conditions Treated
Anxiety, depression, fatigue, headaches, pain, PTSD, stress

Unwanted Effects
Dizziness, dry eyes, dry mouth, paranoia

CINEX

A popular strain that offers clear-headed and uplifting properties, Cinex is a good option for daytime use. It is a great go-to strain for relief from depression and pain.

CANNABINOIDS
THC: 17.80 percent
CBD: 0.19 percent

POTENCY EFFECTS
Creative, energizing, focusing, relaxing, uplifting

Genetic History
Cinderella 99, Vortex

Aroma and Taste
Citrusy, earthy, orange, sweet, skunky

Conditions Treated
Anxiety, arthritis, autoimmune disorders, depression, epilepsy, fatigue, migraines, nausea, pain, PTSD, spasticity, stress

Unwanted Effects
Dizziness, dry eyes, dry mouth, headache, paranoia

DURBAN POISON

This strain hails from Durban, a port city in South Africa. It produces a stimulating, clear-focused, and energetic high, making it ideal for daytime use and exploring the great outdoors.

CANNABINOIDS
THC: 20 percent
THCV: 1 percent
CBD: 0.20 percent
CBG: 1 percent
CBL: 0.30 percent

POTENCY EFFECTS
Creative, energizing, happy, uplifting

Genetic History
African

Aroma and Taste
Earthy, sweet, piney

Conditions Treated
Depression, fatigue, headaches, migraines, stress

Unwanted Effects
Anxiety, dry eyes, dry mouth, paranoia

GREEN CRACK

Rumor has it that this *sativa* was originally called Cush, but after rapper Snoop Dogg experienced its energizing and uplifting effects, he renamed it Green Crack. The unfortunate strain name aside, this *sativa* produces an invigorating, joyful, and focused high, making it a good choice for daytime use. Patients dealing with stress, depression, or fatigue may find this an excellent remedy.

CANNABINOIDS
THC: 20.38 percent
CBD: 0.14 percent

POTENCY EFFECTS
Creative, energizing, euphoric, uplifting

Genetic History
Possibly Skunk #1

Aroma and Taste
Citrusy, earthy, lemon, piney, tropical, spicy

Conditions Treated
Anxiety, depression, fatigue, migraines, nausea, pain, PTSD, stress

Unwanted Effects
Dizziness, dry eyes, dry mouth, headache, paranoia

HARLEQUIN

This CBD-dominant *sativa* is ideal for treating pain and anxiety. It was the first high-CBD strain discovered in the United States and is among the rarest strains. The breeder did not intend to develop a high-CBD strain, but we'll chalk it up to one of those happy accidents.

CANNABINOIDS
THC: 6 percent
THCV: 0.25 percent
CBD: 12 percent
CBG: 0.50 percent

POTENCY EFFECTS
Euphoric, focused, happy, uplifting, relaxing

Genetic History
Colombian Gold, Thai, Swiss *Sativa*

Aroma and Taste
Earthy, piney, woody, sweet

Conditions Treated
Anxiety, depression, gastrointestinal disorders, headaches, inflammation, migraines, nausea, pain, PTSD, stress

Unwanted Effects
Dizziness, dry eyes, dry mouth, headache, paranoia

ISLAND SWEET SKUNK

Island Sweet Skunk is an energizing strain with antianxiety and anti-inflammatory properties. It also helps with nerve pain, migraines, arthritis, and gastrointestinal disorders.

CANNABINOIDS
THC: 20 percent
THCV: 0.05 percent
CBD: 0.01 percent
CBG: 0.10 percent
CBL: 0.04 percent
CBN: 0.03 percent

POTENCY EFFECTS
Energizing, euphoric, happy, uplifting

Genetic History
Skunk #1

Aroma and Taste
Sweet, skunky, tropical

Conditions Treated
Anxiety, arthritis, fatigue, migraines, nausea, pain, PTSD, stress

Unwanted Effects
Anxiety, dry eyes, dry mouth, paranoia

JACK HERER

One of the most award-winning strains in cannabis history, Jack Herer is the namesake of a very influential cannabis activist. It is a classic *sativa* with a clear-headed, creative, and motivating high, making it a great choice for daytime use.

CANNABINOIDS
THC: 19.43 percent
CBD: 0.15 percent
CBG: 1.2 percent

POTENCY EFFECTS
Creative, focused, motivating, upbeat, uplifting

Genetic History
Skunk #1, Northern Lights #5, Haze

Aroma and Taste
Fruity, piney, spicy, skunky

Conditions Treated
Anxiety, arthritis, depression, fatigue, fibromyalgia, lack of focus, migraines, nausea, pain, stress

Unwanted Effects
Dry eyes, dry mouth, paranoia

LAMB'S BREAD

Also known as Lamb's Breath, this energetic and uplifting *sativa* is said to have been one of Bob Marley's favorite strains. It's a great for relieving stress and fighting depression.

- -

CANNABINOIDS

THC: 18 percent
THCV: 0.10 percent
CBD: 0.03 percent
CBG: 0.8 percent

POTENCY EFFECTS

Creative, euphoric, focused, happy, uplifting

- -

Genetic History

Jamaican heritage

Aroma and Taste

Earthy, woody, pungent

Conditions Treated

Depression, fatigue, headaches, migraines, stress

Unwanted Effects

Anxiety, dizziness, dry eyes, dry mouth, paranoia

MAUI WAUI

With its tropical flavors and stress-relieving properties, Maui Waui is reminiscent of being on a Hawaiian vacation. This lightweight *sativa*, which provides energizing, euphoric effects, has been enjoyed since the 1960s. It's also fun to say *mowie-wowie*!

- -

CANNABINOIDS

THC: 18.47 percent
CBD: 0.26 percent

POTENCY EFFECTS

Creative, happy, energetic, euphoric, uplifting

- -

Genetic History

Island *Sativa*, Skunk

Aroma and Taste

Tropical, sweet, citrusy

Conditions Treated

Depression, nausea, pain, stress

Unwanted Effects

Dizziness, dry eyes, dry mouth, headache, paranoia

PURPLE HAZE

Named after Jimi Hendrix's 1967 hit song, this energetic *sativa* produces a creative and euphoric high.

CANNABINOIDS

THC: 20 percent
CBD: 0.06 percent

POTENCY EFFECTS

Energetic, euphoric, happy, relaxing, uplifting

Genetic History

Haze, Purple Thai

Aroma and Taste

Sweet, earthy, berry

Conditions Treated

Depression, insomnia, migraines, pain, stress

Unwanted Effects

Dry eyes, dry mouth, headache, paranoia

SOUR DIESEL

This *sativa* is not only invigorating, but it also produces dreamy cerebral effects. It is a super-pungent strain with a pervasive skunky, lemony scent. It has won four awards, including the 2005 *High Times* Top Ten Strains of the Year.

CANNABINOIDS

THC: 22 percent
CBD: 0.20 percent
CBG: 0.50 percent
CBL: 0.30 percent

POTENCY EFFECTS

Creative, euphoric, energetic, happy, uplifting

Genetic History

Chemdawg, Northern Lights, Skunk

Aroma and Taste

Diesel, earthy, pungent

Conditions Treated

Depression, fatigue, nausea, pain, stress

Unwanted Effects

Dizziness, dry eyes, dry mouth, headache, paranoia

STRAWBERRY COUGH

This sweet *sativa* produces uplifting, euphoric effects, offering relief from anxiety, depression, and stress. Despite its sweet, strawberry flavor, this strain has a tendency to tickle the throat and produce a cough when smoked.

CANNABINOIDS
THC: 19.825 percent
CBD: 0.14 percent

POTENCY EFFECTS
Cerebral, energizing, euphoric, relaxing, uplifting

Genetic History
Strawberry Fields, Original Haze

Aroma and Taste
Berry, strawberry, sweet, skunky

Conditions Treated
Anxiety, lack of appetite, migraines, PTSD, sleep disorders, stress

Unwanted Effects
Dizziness, dry eyes, dry mouth, headache, paranoia

SUPER LEMON HAZE

This 12-time award-winning *sativa* produces a nice balance of both a physical and cerebral high. It has an intense lemony taste followed by an earthy, musky flavor.

CANNABINOIDS
THC: 21.32 percent
CBD: 0.18 percent
CBG: 1.20 percent

POTENCY EFFECTS
Creative, euphoric, relaxing, uplifting

Genetic History
Lemon Skunk, Super Silver Haze

Aroma and Taste
Citrusy, lemony, sweet

Conditions Treated
Anxiety, depression, fatigue, migraines, nausea, pain, stress

Unwanted Effects
Dizziness, dry eyes, dry mouth, paranoia

SUPER SILVER HAZE

A close relative of Jack Herer, this *sativa* is prized for its motivating and energetic properties. It has picked up four awards, including three consecutive years at first place in the *High Times* Cannabis Cup, from 1997 to 1999.

CANNABINOIDS
THC: 20.95 percent
CBD: 0.13 percent

POTENCY EFFECTS
Contemplative, creative, euphoric, energizing, motivating, uplifting

----

Genetic History
Skunk #1, Northern Lights #5, Haze

Aroma and Taste
Citrusy, floral, spicy, sweet

Conditions Treated
Anxiety, arthritis, depression, lack of appetite, migraines, nausea, pain, seizures, stress

Unwanted Effects
Dizziness, dry eyes, dry mouth, headache, paranoia

WILLIE NELSON

This creative, euphoric *sativa* keeps the head clear and mind focused—just what a great singer like Willie Nelson himself might want in a strain. It won the 2005 *High Times* Cannabis Cup in the *sativa* category.

CANNABINOIDS
THC: 18 percent
CBD: 0.14 percent

POTENCY EFFECTS
Creative, euphoric, focusing, happy, uplifting

Genetic History
Heirloom Jamaican strains

Aroma and Taste
Sweet, sour, lemony, earthy, pungent

Conditions Treated
Anxiety, depression, nausea, stress

Unwanted Effects
Dizziness, dry eyes, dry mouth, headache, paranoia

Hybrids began as an attempt to bring out the best of both *indicas* and *sativas*. They are loved by patients who are looking for a blend of *sativa* and *indica* effects. As noted in the previous chapters, researchers continue to find little difference in the effects of *indicas* and *sativas*, and it's unlikely that these classifications will be accurate when discussing hybrids, too. Instead, pay more attention to the available cannabinoid and terpene content of each strain when seeking out the best fit for your symptoms.

HYBRID STRAINS

THIS CHAPTER INCLUDES information on cannabinoid content, taste and aroma, potency effects (both medicinal and recreational), common medicinal uses, and potential unwanted effects (such as dizziness, dry eyes, and dry mouth) of specific hybrid strains. We include the percentage of THC and CBD content for each strain, and when possible, the percentages of other cannabinoids as well. These are average percentages, subject to change based on environmental variations. Just because the percentage of a certain cannabinoid isn't listed, that doesn't mean it's not present in the strain. Unfortunately, cannabinoids other than THC and CBD are still not as well known or tested and therefore are not as available for reporting.

It is also important to understand not only the differences among various strains, but also the potential differences between one strain from two different plants. Environmental factors such as temperature, sunlight, soil type, and nutrients can affect the final output and effects of a plant. While each strain has pretty defined genetics, don't be surprised if O.G. Kush from one grower isn't quite the same as O.G. Kush from another.

Just as in the last chapter, you will notice some bizarre strain names. The names of strains can originate from their appearance, origin, or sometimes even a silly reference created years ago.

ACDC

This high-CBD strain is a *sativa*-dominant hybrid that's related to Cannatonic. With a 1:20 THC to CBD ratio, it has no psychoactive effects.

CANNABINOIDS
THC: 1.35 percent
CBD: 24.97 percent
CBG: 0.20 percent

POTENCY EFFECTS
Focusing, relaxing, social, upbeat

Genetic History
MK Ultra, G13 Haze

Aroma and Taste
Earthy, citrusy, lemony, woody

Conditions Treated
Anxiety, cancer, depression, epilepsy, inflammation, multiple sclerosis, pain, PTSD, stress

Unwanted Effects
Dizziness, dry eyes, dry mouth

AGENT ORANGE

This uplifting and flavorful *sativa*-dominant hybrid is ideal for combatting fatigue and depression. With its sweet, citrusy flavor, it is considered by many to be one of the best-tasting strains.

CANNABINOIDS
THC: 19 percent
CBD: 0.14 percent

POTENCY EFFECTS
Euphoric, energizing, happy, relaxed, uplifting

Genetic History
Orange Velvet, Jack the Ripper

Aroma and Taste
Citrusy, orange, sour

Conditions Treated
Depression, fatigue, headache, nausea, stress

Unwanted Effects
Dry eyes, dry mouth, paranoia

BLUE DREAM

A great-tasting hybrid, Blue Dream produces full-body relaxation with a calm euphoria. Originating in California, it is increasingly popular on the West Coast.

- -

CANNABINOIDS
THC: 21.84 percent
CBD: 0.21 percent

POTENCY EFFECTS
Cerebral, creative, energizing, euphoric, focusing, relaxing, uplifting

- -

Genetic History
Blueberry, Haze

Aroma and Taste
Berry, blueberry, spicy, sweet

Conditions Treated
Anorexia, depression, migraines, nausea, pain, sleep disorders, stress

Unwanted Effects
Dry eyes, dry mouth

CANNATONIC

This popular hybrid has a 1:1 ratio of THC to CBD, providing an uplifting high with minimal psychoactive effects. It placed third in its category in the 2008 *High Times* Cannabis Cup.

- -

CANNABINOIDS
THC: 8.21 percent
CBD: 8.33 percent

POTENCY EFFECTS
Creative, euphoric, social, uplifting

- -

Genetic History
MK Ultra, G13 Haze

Aroma and Taste
Earthy, piney, citrusy, lemony

Conditions Treated
Arthritis, depression, headache, inflammation, nausea, migraines, pain

Unwanted Effects
Dry eyes, dry mouth

CHARLOTTE'S WEB

This CBD-dominant hybrid is famous for its ability to help relieve epilepsy and seizures. Despite bearing the title of the popular children's book, it was named for Charlotte Figi, a young girl with intractable epilepsy whose disorder was successfully treated with CBD-rich cannabis. She went from being wheelchair-bound and having over 300 seizures a week to being largely seizure-free and walking. Her story has spurred legalization of CBD-only marijuana in states without medical marijuana programs.

- -

CANNABINOIDS
THC: 0.92 percent
CBD: 16.86 percent

POTENCY EFFECTS
Energizing, focusing,
relaxing, uplifting

- -

Genetic History
Unknown marijuana strain
crossed with an industrial
hemp strain

Aroma and Taste
Earthy, floral, piney

Conditions Treated
Depression, epilepsy, pain,
seizures, spasticity, stress

Unwanted Effects
Anxiety, dizziness,
dry eyes, headache

CHEMDAWG

This strain has won four awards, including first place at the 2012 Emerald Cup. As the legend goes, a man by the name of Chemdog purchased this strain with seeds at a Grateful Dead concert; the plant was cultivated, producing the Chemdawg we know and love today.

- -

CANNABINOIDS
THC: 22 percent
CBD: 0.5 percent
CBG: 1 percent

POTENCY EFFECTS
Creative, euphoric,
relaxing, uplifting

- -

Genetic History
Unknown

Aroma and Taste
Earthy, pungent, diesel

Conditions Treated
Depression, insomnia,
nausea, pain, stress

Unwanted Effects
Dizziness, dry eyes, dry mouth

GIRL SCOUT COOKIES

Taking home a prize in several Cannabis Cups, this *indica*-dominant hybrid brings on a strong, relaxing, and therapeutic high.

CANNABINOIDS
THC: 21.23 percent
CBD: 0.17 percent

POTENCY EFFECTS
Creative, euphoric, relaxing, social, uplifting

Genetic History
Possibly O.G. Kush, Durban Poison, Cherry Kush

Aroma and Taste
Earthy, fruity, floral, piney

Conditions Treated
Anxiety, arthritis, headaches, inflammation, lack of appetite, migraines, multiple sclerosis, nausea, pain, Parkinson's disease, sleep disorders, spinal cord injury, stress

Unwanted Effects
Dry eyes, dry mouth

GREAT WHITE SHARK

Also known as Peacemaker, this winner of seven awards produces a pleasant and potent head and body high.

CANNABINOIDS
THC: 15.63 percent
CBD: 0.11 percent

POTENCY EFFECTS
Energizing, euphoric, uplifting

Genetic History
White Widow, Skunk #1

Aroma and Taste
Earthy, fruity, sweet

Conditions Treated
Depression, gastrointestinal disorders, nausea, pain, PMS

Unwanted Effects
Dry eyes, dry mouth, paranoia

HARLE-TSU

A CBD-dominant hybrid with a THC to CBD ratio of 1:20, Harle-Tsu is great for relieving pain and inflammation without psychoactive effects. This strain placed first in the 2012 and 2013 Emerald Cup for the highest CBD content.

CANNABINOIDS

THC: 6.40 percent
CBD: 9.65 percent

POTENCY EFFECTS

Energizing, euphoric, focusing, giggly, relaxing

Genetic History

Sour Tsunami, Harlequin

Aroma and Taste

Earthy, lemony, fuel, piney, woody

Conditions Treated

Fibromyalgia, inflammation, sleep disorders, spinal cord injury

Unwanted Effects

Dizziness, dry mouth

ICE

A first-place winner in the 1998 *High Times* Cannabis Cup, Ice is an *indica*-dominant strain named for its abundance of dense trichomes. It produces a heavy, sedating body high.

CANNABINOIDS

THC: 16.89 percent
CBD: 0.20 percent

POTENCY EFFECTS

Euphoric, giggly, relaxing, sleep-inducing

Genetic History

Afghani, Skunk #1, Northern Lights

Aroma and Taste

Skunky, earthy, sweet

Conditions Treated

Anxiety, arthritis, depression, lack of appetite, pain, PTSD, sleep disorders, spinal cord injury, seizures, stress, Tourette syndrome

Unwanted Effects

Dry eyes, dry mouth

O.G. KUSH

This popular medical strain is extremely potent. There is some debate about what "O.G." stands for; some say "Ocean Grown" due to its California origins, while others say "Original Gangster," which is another cannabis strain. Regardless of its origins, this well-known, popular strain is one of the most common hybrids on the market.

CANNABINOIDS
THC: 15 percent
CBD: 0.01 percent

POTENCY EFFECTS
Euphoric, narcotic, relaxing, uplifting

Genetic History
Chemdawg, Hindu Kush, Lemon Thai

Aroma and Taste
Earthy, lemony, fuel, spicy, sweet, piney, woody

Conditions Treated
Alzheimer's disease, anxiety, arthritis, depression, fibromyalgia, glaucoma, headaches, migraines, multiple sclerosis, pain, PMS, PTSD, seizures, stress

Unwanted Effects
Dry eyes, dry mouth

PERMA FROST

Named for its thick, glorious coating of resin, this *sativa*-dominant hybrid produces euphoric and uplifting effects, making it great for daytime use.

CANNABINOIDS
THC: 19 percent
CBD: 0.15 percent

POTENCY EFFECTS
Creative, euphoric, happy, relaxing

Genetic History
White Widow, Trainwreck

Aroma and Taste
Earthy, floral, fruity, piney, spicy, sweet

Conditions Treated
Anxiety, depression, fibromyalgia, gastrointestinal disorders, headaches, insomnia, lack of appetite, migraines, nausea, pain, spasticity, stress

Unwanted Effects
Dry eyes, dry mouth

PIT BULL

Pit Bull is a relaxing hybrid that's great for pain and stress relief. Like its namesake, this strain is hardy with an instinct for survival, making it an ideal plant for new growers.

- -

CANNABINOIDS
THC: 18.69 percent
CBD: 0.11 percent

POTENCY EFFECTS
Focusing, social, upbeat

- -

Genetic History
Sugar Plum, P91

Aroma and Taste
Fruity, tropical, skunky, earthy

Conditions Treated
Cancer, cramps, depression, glaucoma, HIV, AIDS, lack of appetite, migraines, multiple sclerosis, nausea, neuropathy, pain, sleep disorders

Unwanted Effects
Dry eyes, dry mouth

REMEDY

Finally, a strain name with a medicinal meaning! This relaxing CBD-dominant strain has wonderful health benefits with virtually no psychoactive effects.

- -

CANNABINOIDS
THC: 0.84 percent
CBD: 12.83 percent

POTENCY EFFECTS
Focusing, relaxing, sleep-inducing

- -

Genetic History
Cannatonic, Afghan, Skunk

Aroma and Taste
Earthy, floral, lemony, piney

Conditions Treated
Anxiety, epilepsy, hypertension, migraines, pain, PTSD, sleep disorders, spasticity, stress

Unwanted Effects
Dry eyes, dry mouth

SKYWALKER

Skywalker is an easygoing, *indica*-dominant hybrid that perhaps would have mellowed out even Darth Vader. It has powerful, pain-relieving properties along with a sedating, relaxing body high that isn't overly hazy.

- -

CANNABINOIDS
THC: 18.50 percent
CBD: 0.22 percent

POTENCY EFFECTS
Euphoric, relaxing, sedating, sleep-inducing

- -

Genetic History
Blueberry, Mazar

Aroma and Taste
Earthy, fruity, sweet

Conditions Treated
Anxiety, arthritis, depression, lack of appetite, migraines, nausea, pain, spinal cord injury, stress

Unwanted Effects
Dizziness, dry mouth, headache, paranoia

SOUR TSUNAMI

An award-winning, CBD-dominant hybrid, Sour Tsunami targets pain and inflammation-related disorders. It was one of the first strains to be bred specifically for a high level of CBD.

- -

CANNABINOIDS
THC: 0.85 percent
CBD: 14.27 percent

POTENCY EFFECTS
Focusing, happy, relaxing, sleep-inducing

- -

Genetic History
Sour Diesel, NYC Diesel, Ferrari

Aroma and Taste
Earthy, musky, fuel, piney, sweet

Conditions Treated
Anxiety, arthritis, cancer, depression, gastrointestinal disorders, inflammation, pain, spasticity, stress

Unwanted Effects
Anxiety, dry eyes, dry mouth, paranoia

TRAINWRECK

This potent, *sativa*-dominant hybrid is sought for its powerful cerebral high and deep body relaxation. The name came about, supposedly, when two brothers were forced to harvest their cannabis plants early due to a nearby train wreck. Fortunately, the crop was ready earlier than most other *sativa* breeds and the name stuck.

CANNABINOIDS
THC: 18.18 percent
CBD: 0.19 percent

POTENCY EFFECTS
Creative, euphoric, relaxing, uplifting

Genetic History
Possibly Lowland Thai, Mexican Sativa, Afghani

Aroma and Taste
Berry, earthy, fruity, lemony, piney, spicy

Conditions Treated
Anxiety, arthritis, depression, headache, migraines, pain, PTSD, sleep disorders, stress

Unwanted Effects
Dry eyes, dry mouth

WHITE WIDOW

White Widow brings on a spacey, powerful high that can produce paranoia and lethargy, so it might not be for everyone. This resin-coated strain took home first place in the 1995 *High Times* Cannabis Cup, after just entering the market in 1994.

CANNABINOIDS
THC: 19.24 percent
CBD: 0.15 percent

POTENCY EFFECTS
Creative, euphoric, psychedelic, relaxing, social, uplifting

Genetic History
Indian Kush, Brazilian Sativa

Aroma and Taste
Earthy, fruity, floral, piney

Conditions Treated
Anxiety, depression, migraines, nausea, pain, PMS, sleep disorders, stress

Unwanted Effects
Anxiety, dry eyes, dry mouth, lethargy, paranoia

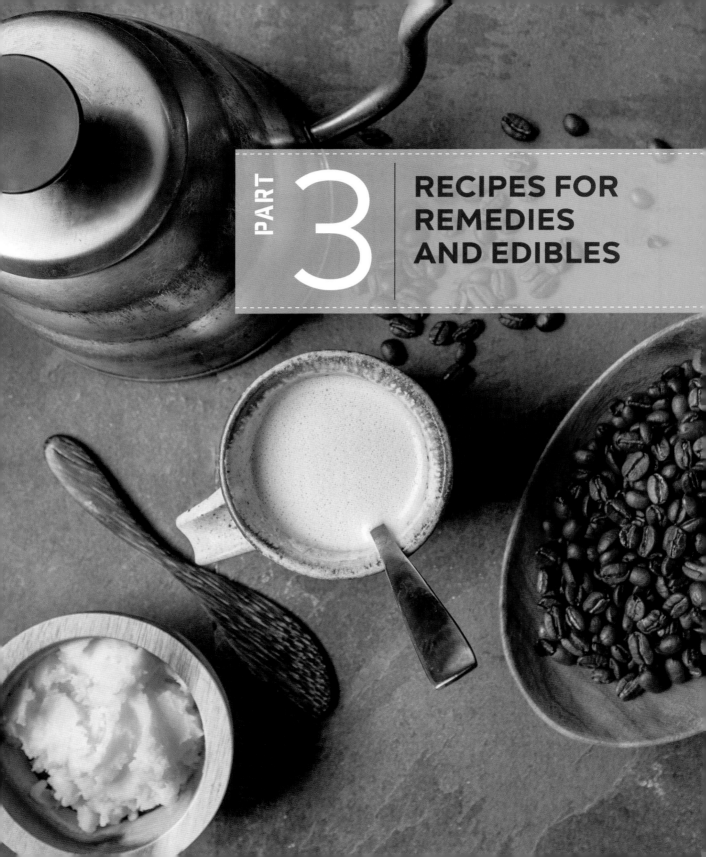

PART 3 RECIPES FOR REMEDIES AND EDIBLES

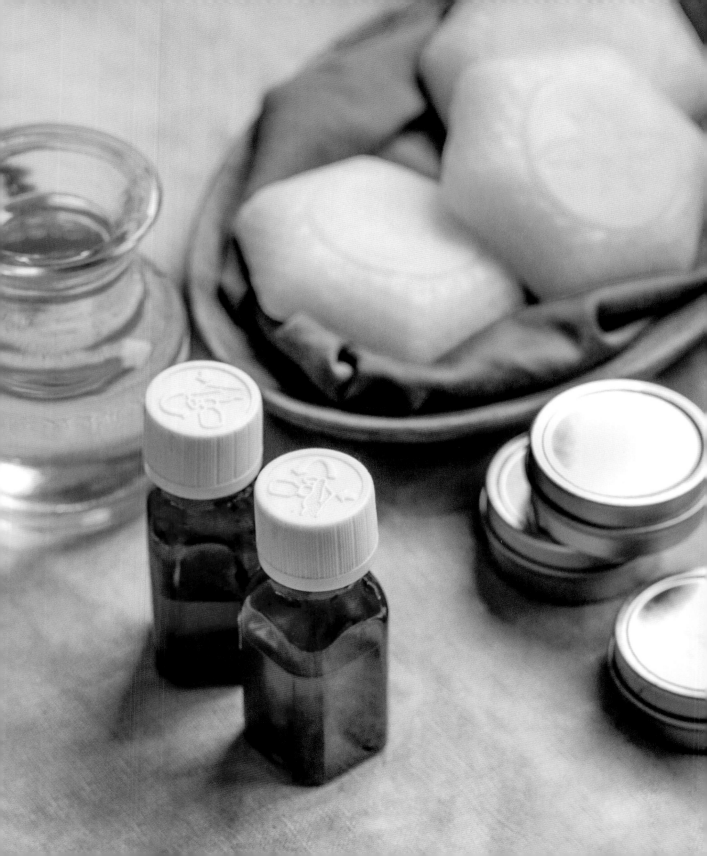

CANNABIS REMEDIES

CANNABIS TREATMENTS AND delivery methods extend well beyond just smoking the flower. However, even if you have access to a dispensary, some of these options— including edibles, capsules, tinctures, suppositories, and topicals—can be hard to find and are often a little pricey. By making these remedies at home, you can ensure quality, consistency, accessibility, and affordability.

Most of the ingredients in these recipes (aside from the cannabis, of course) can be found at your local grocery store. For special ingredients, such as glycerin and essential oils, look online or in your local health food store.

Required Equipment

Blender—This kitchen appliance is used to blend, purée, liquefy, and emulsify. You can use a standard blender or an immersion blender. You can find a blender online or at your local kitchen and home supply store.

Candy molds—Candy molds, which come in various shapes and sizes, are used to form candy into consistently sized pieces. You can find candy molds online or at your local kitchen and home supply store, as well as at your local craft store.

Candy thermometer—This kitchen thermometer is capable of withstanding high heat. You can find one online or at your local kitchen and home supply store.

Capsule-filling machine—This mechanical device enables you to fill many capsules at once. Capsules can be filled by hand, but a filling machine makes the work easier and more efficient. You can find a capsule-filling machine online or at your local naturopathic health store.

Capsules, empty (size 00)—Empty capsules are small shells with two parts that fit together to hold medicine. They are usually made of gelatin, but vegan alternatives are available. You can find them online or at your local naturopathic health store.

Cheesecloth—This loosely woven cloth is traditionally used for making cheese, but it's also good for straining liquids. You can find cheesecloth online or at your local kitchen and home supply store.

Coffee grinder or food processor—A coffee grinder is a small kitchen appliance that quickly processes dry ingredients into a fine powder. A food processor can be used for the same purpose, but a coffee grinder is perfect for small amounts. You can find a coffee grinder or food processor online or at your local kitchen and home supply store.

Fine mesh strainer—This is a handled, metal mesh bowl through which you can strain liquids. Look for one that will sit on top of a bowl without falling in for mess-free straining. You can find a strainer online or at your local kitchen and home supply store.

Sifter—A sifter is used to separate and break up clumps in dry ingredients, usually flour. It also aerates the ingredients, and when more than one ingredient is used, it helps to combine them more evenly. You can find a sifter online or at your local kitchen and home supply store.

Suppository molds (2.3-milliliter)—Molds for making suppositories are generally bullet-shaped and may be plastic, rubber, or metal. You can find suppository molds online.

Syringe with tapered tip—Used for filling capsules, a syringe with a tapered tip allows for precise application. You can find a syringe with a tapered tip online.

CANNA-OIL

GLUTEN-FREE | NUT-FREE | SOY-FREE | SUGAR-FREE | VEGAN

Prized for its many health benefits, coconut oil can be used as a base for a wide variety of edibles and topicals. Although coconut oil is used in this recipe, you can swap it out for your preferred oil, such as olive oil, sesame oil, canola oil, or vegetable oil.

MAKES 28 OUNCES
[1 teaspoon = 1 serving]
Prep time: 5 minutes
Cook time: 4 hours

Required Equipment
Cheesecloth
Fine mesh strainer

 DOSAGE TEST

Start with ¼ teaspoon of canna-oil and wait 4 hours to fully assess your reaction to its strength and effects.

14 grams cannabis
28 ounces coconut oil

1. Preheat the oven to 240°F.

2. Place the cannabis on a rimmed baking sheet and bake for 45 minutes to activate the THC, resulting in decarboxylated cannabis.

3. In a medium saucepan, heat the oil over low heat until melted.

4. Add the decarboxylated cannabis to the oil. Stir to mix.

5. Continue to cook for 3 hours over low heat, stirring occasionally. The oil should not boil or simmer, although it may bubble occasionally.

6. Line a fine mesh strainer with cheesecloth and place it over a large, heat-safe bowl. Carefully pour the oil through the cheesecloth, allowing any excess oil to strain through.

7. Remove the cheesecloth from the strainer, using gloves if the oil is still very hot, and squeeze any remaining oil into the bowl.

8. Allow the oil to cool slightly before transferring to an airtight container. The shelf life of your canna-oil depends on the base oil you used; canna-oil made with coconut oil lasts up to 1 year.

- -

In our kitchen, we cook with cannabis that has 15 percent THC, which results in 10 milligrams of THC per teaspoon of canna-oil. If you need a higher or lower dose, you can either use more or less cannabis when making your canna-oil or increase or decrease the amount of oil called for in a recipe.

PER SERVING Calories: 39; Total Fat: 4.5g; Saturated Fat: 3.9g; Cholesterol: 0mg; Carbohydrates: 0g; Fiber: 0g; Protein: 0g

CANNA-BUTTER

GLUTEN-FREE | NUT-FREE | SOY-FREE | SUGAR-FREE | VEGETARIAN

Canna-butter is a well-loved classic in the cannabis world. It provides a wonderful base to make a range of delicious edible creations. To avoid the need to skim off the milk solids, you can use 28 ounces (1¾ pounds) of clarified butter, or ghee, instead of the unsalted butter. If you decide to vary the amounts of your ingredients, just be sure that the cannabis is always floating 1½ to 2 inches from the bottom of the pan.

MAKES 28 OUNCES

[1 teaspoon = 1 serving]
Prep time: 5 minutes
Cook time: 4 hours

Required Equipment
Cheesecloth
Fine mesh strainer

 DOSAGE TEST

Start with ¼ teaspoon of canna-butter and wait 4 hours to fully assess your reaction to its strength and effects.

14 grams cannabis
4 cups water
2 pounds (8 sticks) unsalted butter

1. Preheat the oven to 240ºF.

2. Place the cannabis on a rimmed baking sheet and bake for 45 minutes to activate the THC, resulting in decarboxylated cannabis.

3. In a medium saucepan, bring the water to a boil.

4. Add the butter and continue to heat until the butter is completely melted. Skim off the milk solids that rise to the surface.

5. Turn the heat to low, and add the decarboxylated cannabis. The cannabis should float 1½ to 2 inches from the bottom of the pan.

6. Cook for 3 hours at a very low simmer, stirring occasionally.

7. Line a fine mesh strainer with cheesecloth and place it over a large, heat-safe bowl. Carefully pour the butter through the cheesecloth, allowing the butter to strain through.

8. Remove the cheesecloth from the strainer, using gloves if the butter is still hot, and squeeze any remaining butter into the bowl.

9. Allow the butter to cool slightly before transferring to an airtight container. Store in the refrigerator about 1 week.

- -

In our kitchen, we cook with cannabis that has 15 percent THC, which results in 10 milligrams of THC per teaspoon of canna-butter. If you need a higher or lower dose, you can either use more or less cannabis when making your canna-butter.

PER SERVING Calories: 45; Total Fat: 5g; Saturated Fat: 3g; Cholesterol: 11mg; Carbohydrates: 0g; Fiber: 0g; Protein: 0g

CANNA-FLOUR

GLUTEN-FREE | NUT-FREE | SOY-FREE | SUGAR-FREE | VEGAN

Unlike infused butter and oil, canna-flour involves cooking with and consuming the whole plant. Not only is it a fiber boost and loaded with great nutrients and medicine, it's super simple to prepare. The only downside is the taste—if you have an aversion to the taste of cannabis, this might not be the method for you.

MAKES ¼ CUP

Prep time: 5 minutes
Cook time: 45 minutes

Required Equipment
Food processor
   or coffee grinder
Sifter

 DOSAGE TEST

Start with one-fourth of a serving of the edibles you prepare with canna-flour and wait 4 hours to fully assess your reaction to its strength and effects.

7 grams cannabis

1. Preheat the oven to 240ºF.

2. Place the cannabis on a rimmed baking sheet and bake for 45 minutes to activate the THC, resulting in decarboxylated cannabis. Allow to cool.

3. Transfer the decarboxylated cannabis to a food processor or coffee grinder. Process the cannabis into a very fine powder.

4. Transfer the canna-flour to an airtight container and store in a cool, dark, dry place until ready to use. Use within 3 months for optimal freshness.

- -

Replace up to one-fourth of the amount of flour called for in a recipe with this canna-flour. Sift the flour and canna-flour together to blend evenly prior to use to ensure consistent dosing in your baked goods. When baking with canna-flour, do not exceed temperatures of 340ºF. Cannabis has a strong flavor, so you may want to increase other strong flavors in your baked item to balance it out. ■ In our kitchen, we cook with cannabis that has 15 percent THC, which results in 10 milligrams of THC per teaspoon of canna-flour. You may want to use more or less cannabis depending on your dosage level and the number of servings in your prepared dish.

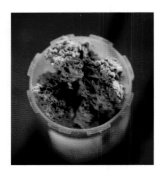

THOUGHTS AND EXPERIENCES

Three years ago, I began studying the medicinal benefits of cannabis. It was simple curiosity until my friend—a vibrant, healthy individual—was diagnosed with lymphoma. I immediately had to learn if cannabis could help destroy this horrendous disease.

Long story short, my friend now uses high-CBD full-extract oil daily. The oil arrested and destroyed the cancer! Oregon's Finest, the dispensary where I work, connected my friend to an amazing grower who supplies the oil and provides support for preventive treatment.

After witnessing the benefits, I decided to try it myself. I've struggled with irritable bowel syndrome (IBS) for as long as I can recall. Gastroenterologists can't explain the symptoms, and I was on a variety of meds. If the meds were not taken religiously, they had no beneficial effect and they caused unpleasant side effects like vertigo. I first tried cannabis for my IBS about two years ago and found that a few drops of high-CBD tincture or a few puffs of a sativa-dominant strain immediately relieved painful cramps.

I feel lucky to be involved in the cannabis industry, and I cannot wait to see what more is discovered! —**S.S.**, Oregon's Finest employee and patient, Portland, Oregon

CANNA-CAPSULES

GLUTEN-FREE | NUT-FREE | SOY-FREE | SUGAR-FREE | VEGAN

Canna-capsules are an easy and consistent way to enjoy the effects of edibles in pill form. There is a small start-up cost involved in making canna-capsules. You will need a capsule-filling machine, perhaps a syringe, and size 00 empty capsules. Capsules are usually made with gelatin, but vegetable-based alternatives are also available.

MAKES 200 CAPSULES

Prep time: 5 minutes
Cook time: 4 hours

Required Equipment
Fine mesh strainer
Cheesecloth
Size 00 empty capsules
Capsule-filling machine
10-milliliter syringe with
   tapered tip

 DOSAGE TEST

Start with 1 canna-capsule and wait 4 hours to fully assess your reaction to its strength and effects.

8 grams cannabis
7 ounces coconut oil

1. Preheat the oven to 240°F.

2. Place the cannabis on a rimmed baking sheet and bake for 45 minutes to activate the THC, resulting in decarboxylated cannabis.

3. In a small saucepan, heat the coconut oil over low heat. Add the decarboxylated cannabis to the oil. Stir to mix.

4. Cook for 3 hours over low heat, stirring occasionally. The oil should not boil or simmer, although it may bubble occasionally.

5. Line a fine mesh strainer with cheesecloth and place it over a large, heat-safe bowl. Carefully pour the oil through the cheesecloth, allowing any excess oil to strain through.

6. Remove the cheesecloth from the strainer, using gloves if the oil is still very hot, and squeeze any remaining oil into the bowl.

7. Follow the directions on the capsule-filling machine. While the oil is still in liquid form, fill the capsules using a syringe with a tapered tip, if necessary. If the oil solidifies before filling the capsules, reheat over low heat.

8. Store the capsules in an airtight container in the refrigerator for up to 1 year.

- -

It is advisable to take a canna-capsule with a little bit of food—not on a completely empty stomach, but not on a full stomach either. ■ *In our kitchen, we cook with cannabis that has 15 percent THC, which results in 5 milligrams of THC per canna-capsule. If you need a higher or lower dose, you can use more or less cannabis when making your canna-capsules.*

CANNA-SIMPLE SYRUP

GLUTEN-FREE | NUT-FREE | SOY-FREE | VEGAN

This simple syrup is a wonderful way to infuse drinks, desserts, and candies. It is a relatively quick infusion, requiring just about 30 minutes on the stove.

MAKES 24 OUNCES

[2 tablespoons = 1 serving]
Prep time: 5 minutes
Cook time: 1 hour, 15 minutes

Required Equipment
Cheesecloth
Fine mesh strainer

 DOSAGE TEST

Start with 2 teaspoons of canna-simple syrup and wait 4 hours to fully assess your reaction to its strength and effects.

4 grams cannabis, coarsely ground
3 cups water
3 cups granulated sugar
3 tablespoons vegetable glycerin

1. Preheat the oven to 240ºF.

2. Place the cannabis on a rimmed baking sheet and bake for 45 minutes to activate the THC, resulting in decarboxylated cannabis.

3. In a medium saucepan, combine the water and sugar, and bring to a low boil over medium heat.

4. Add the decarboxylated cannabis and cover the saucepan. Cook for 20 minutes.

5. Add the glycerin and reduce the heat. Simmer for 7 to 8 minutes, stirring occasionally. The mixture will thicken.

6. Line a fine mesh strainer with cheesecloth and place it over a large, heat-safe bowl. Carefully pour the syrup through the cheesecloth.

7. Remove the cheesecloth from the strainer, using gloves if the syrup is still very hot, and squeeze any remaining syrup into the bowl.

8. Allow the syrup to cool slightly before transferring to an airtight container. Store in the refrigerator for up to 3 weeks.

- -

In our kitchen, we cook with cannabis that has 15 percent THC, which results in 10 milligrams of THC per 2 tablespoons of this syrup. If you need a higher or lower dose, you can use more or less cannabis when making this recipe.

PER SERVING Calories: 104; Total Fat: 0g; Saturated Fat: 0g; Cholesterol: 0mg; Carbohydrates: 28g; Fiber: 0g; Protein: 0g

HERBAL CANNABIS TEA

GLUTEN-FREE | NUT-FREE | SOY-FREE | SUGAR-FREE | VEGAN

In his encyclopedic work, Naturalis Historia (77–79 CE), Pliny the Elder described boiling the cannabis root in water to make a tea that relieves joint pain. Today, the roots and stems are still used to make this infusion. If you grow your own cannabis, save the stems and roots of the plants after harvest. This tea has virtually zero psychoactive effects because the stems contain low levels of cannabinoids; they do, however, contain beneficial terpenes that can help reduce inflammation and pain.

MAKES 80 OUNCES

[8 ounces = 1 serving]
Prep time: 10 minutes
Cook time: 1 hour, plus
    overnight steeping

Required Equipment
Cheesecloth
Fine mesh strainer

 DOSAGE TEST

Start with half of a serving and wait 4 hours to fully assess your reaction to its strength and effects.

10 cups water
Stems and roots from 1 cannabis plant, dried and roughly chopped
3 herbal teabags (any type)

1. In a large saucepan, bring the water to a boil.

2. Reduce the heat to low and add the chopped stems and roots. Cover and cook for 1 hour.

3. Remove from the heat and add the herbal teabags. Cover and steep overnight on the countertop.

4. Line a fine mesh strainer with cheesecloth and place it over a bowl.

5. Carefully pour the tea through the cheesecloth. Gently press to extract any remaining tea water through the cheesecloth.

6. Serve warm or cold.

7. Store the remaining servings in a pitcher in the refrigerator as you would any other iced tea.

- -

You can leave the herbal tea out of this recipe for plain cannabis tea. ■ *The cannabis root contains alkaloids that can cause liver damage if consumed in high amounts or for a long period of time. This herbal tea should be limited to 1 cup a day with light to moderate long-term use.*

CANNABIS BHANG TEA

GLUTEN-FREE | SOY-FREE | VEGETARIAN

Bhang is a cannabis-infused tea served during the Hindu festival of Holi each year. This is one of the oldest known methods of ingesting canna- bis. Depending on the strain you use, this heavily spiced and creamy tea may make you melt into your seat or send you dancing.

MAKES 48 OUNCES

[8 ounces = 1 serving]
Prep time: 15 minutes
Cook time: 1 hour, 30 minutes

Required Equipment
Cheesecloth
Fine mesh strainer

 DOSAGE TEST

Start with half of a serving and wait 4 hours to fully assess your reaction to its strength and effects.

8 grams cannabis, coarsely ground
2 cups water
1 tablespoon unsalted butter
4 cups whole milk
2 tablespoons almond flour
¼ teaspoon garam masala
2 teaspoons loose chai tea
½ cup honey
Half-and-half or cream

1. Preheat the oven to 240°F.

2. Place the cannabis on a rimmed baking sheet and bake for 45 minutes to activate the THC, resulting in decarboxylated cannabis.

3. In a medium saucepan, bring the water, butter, and milk to a boil.

4. Reduce the heat to low, and add the decarboxylated canna- bis, almond flour, and garam masala. Cover and simmer for 30 to 45 minutes.

5. Remove from the heat and add the tea to the saucepan. Steep for 7 minutes.

6. Line a fine mesh strainer with cheesecloth and place it over a large, heat-safe bowl. Carefully pour the tea through the cheesecloth. Press to extract any remaining liquid through the cheesecloth.

7. Add the honey to the bowl and stir until dissolved.

8. Pour the tea into a mug and add the desired amount of half-and-half or cream.

9. Store the remaining servings in an airtight container in the refrigerator for up to 1 week. To reheat, heat in a small saucepan over low heat.

- -

To simplify the preparation, use 2 tablespoons of canna-butter (page 106) in place of the cannabis and butter and reduce the simmering time to 15 minutes. ■ *In our kitchen, we cook with cannabis that has 15 percent THC, which results in 10 milligrams of THC per 8-ounce serving of this tea. If you need a higher or lower dose, you can use more or less cannabis when making this recipe.*

PER SERVING
without half-and-half or cream: Calories: 238; Total Fat: 9.9g; Saturated Fat: 3.5g; Cholesterol: 18mg; Carbohydrates: 33.3g; Fiber: 1.1g; Protein: 7.4g

CANNA-COFFEE

GLUTEN-FREE | NUT-FREE | SOY-FREE | SUGAR-FREE | VEGETARIAN

Canna-coffee is the way to go if you need to medicate in the morning. It is as simple as blending some canna-butter or canna-oil (for a vegan alternative) with your brewed coffee for a creamy, soothing drink. It doesn't matter if the coffee is caffeinated or decaf. This method works well with tea, too.

MAKES 1 SERVING

Prep time: 10 minutes

Required Equipment
Immersion blender

 DOSAGE TEST

Start with ¼ teaspoon of canna-butter or canna-oil in your coffee and wait 4 hours to fully assess your reaction to its strength and effects.

1 teaspoon canna-butter (page 106) or canna-oil (page 105)
1 tablespoon butter or coconut oil
1 cup brewed coffee, hot
Sweetener (optional)

1. Using an immersion blender, blend the butters or oils into the coffee for about 30 seconds until creamy and frothy.

2. Pour into a cup and add sweetener, if using.

3. Serve immediately.

- -

If you are on a low-fat diet, you can use cannabis tincture (page 119) for 10 milligrams of THC in place of the canna-butter or canna-oil, or simply omit the additional tablespoon of butter or oil.

PER SERVING
with butter: Calories: 151; Total Fat: 17g; Saturated Fat: 11g; Cholesterol: 45mg; Carbohydrates: 0g; Fiber: 0g; Protein: 0.2g
with coconut oil: Calories: 181; Total Fat: 21g; Saturated Fat: 18g; Cholesterol: 0mg; Carbohydrates: 0g; Fiber: 0g; Protein: 0g

CANNA-CIDER

GLUTEN-FREE | NUT-FREE | SOY-FREE | VEGETARIAN

Hot spiced cider is such a soothing and uplifting cold-weather treat. Apple cider itself boasts a number of important health bene-fits: it is a great source of antioxidants, helps prevent asthma, cleanses the liver, reduces cholesterol, boosts the immune system, and may even help prevent cancer. In tandem with a cannabis infusion, this dose of medicine will work like a charm.

MAKES 16 OUNCES
[8 ounces = 1 serving]
Prep time: 10 minutes
Cook time: 10 minutes

 DOSAGE TEST

Start with half of a serving of canna-cider and wait 4 hours to fully assess your reaction to its strength and effects.

2 cups apple cider
1 tablespoon honey
1 cinnamon stick
1 orange peel
2 whole cloves
1 whole star anise
2 teaspoons canna-butter (page 106) or
    1 teaspoon cannabis tincture (page 119)

1. In a small saucepan, bring the cider, honey, cinnamon stick, orange peel, cloves, and star anise to a boil.

2. Reduce the heat, cover, and simmer for 10 minutes. Remove from the heat.

3. Using a slotted spoon, remove the cinnamon stick, orange peel, cloves, and star anise from the liquid.

4. Add the canna-butter or tincture to the liquid, and stir well.

5. Pour into mugs and serve warm.

6. Store the remaining serving in an airtight container in the refrigerator for up to 1 week. To reheat, heat in a small saucepan over low heat.

- -

Homemade apple cider is a treat in this recipe. To get 2 cups of fresh-pressed cider, juice 3 or 4 apples.

PER SERVING
with canna-butter: Calories: 182; Total Fat: 4.1g; Saturated Fat: 2.5g; Cholesterol: 10mg; Carbohydrates: 37.6g; Fiber: 0g; Protein: 0.2g
with cannabis tincture: Calories: 148; Total Fat: 0.3g; Saturated Fat: 0g; Cholesterol: 0mg; Carbohydrates: 37.6g; Fiber: 0g; Protein: 0.2g

HOT SPICED ORANGE JUICE
WITH CANNABIS

GLUTEN-FREE | NUT-FREE | SOY-FREE | VEGETARIAN

This warm, citrusy beverage hits the spot during cold and flu season. It is soothing, nourishing, and filled with immune-boosting nutrients to help bring you back to health.

MAKES 16 OUNCES

[8 ounces = 1 serving]
Prep time: 10 minutes
Cook time: 5 minutes

 DOSAGE TEST

Start with half of a serving of hot spiced orange juice and wait 4 hours to fully assess your reaction to its strength and effects.

1½ cups freshly squeezed orange juice
½ cup water
1 teaspoon freshly grated or ground ginger
⅛ teaspoon ground cinnamon
⅛ teaspoon ground turmeric
2 tablespoons honey
2 teaspoons canna-oil (page 105) or
    1 teaspoon cannabis tincture (page 119)

1. In a small saucepan, combine the orange juice, water, ginger, cinnamon, and turmeric. Bring to a low simmer.

2. Reduce the heat, cover, and warm for 5 minutes.

3. Remove from the heat and stir in the honey and canna-oil or cannabis tincture.

4. Pour into mugs and serve warm.

5. Store the remaining serving in an airtight container in the refrigerator for up to 5 days. To reheat, heat in a small saucepan over low heat.

- -

For a nutrient boost, replace the water with an equal amount of prune juice or pomegranate juice.

PER SERVING
with canna-oil: Calories: 187; Total Fat: 4.9g; Saturated Fat: 4g; Cholesterol: 0mg; Carbohydrates: 36.7g; Fiber: 0g; Protein: 1.3g
with cannabis tincture: Calories: 148; Total Fat: 0.4g; Saturated Fat: 0g; Cholesterol: 0mg; Carbohydrates: 36.7g; Fiber: 0g; Protein: 1.3g

GOLDEN MILK

GLUTEN-FREE | NUT-FREE | SOY-FREE | VEGETARIAN

Turmeric is packed with anti-oxidant, anti-inflammatory, immune-boosting nutrients. Golden milk is a wonderful and delicious way to take in turmeric and a host of other nourishing spices. Its relaxing properties also make this a delightful nighttime drink.

MAKES 24 OUNCES

[8 ounces = 1 serving]
Prep time: 10 minutes
Cook time: 5 minutes

Required Equipment
Immersion blender

 DOSAGE TEST

Start with half of a serving of golden milk and wait 4 hours to fully assess your reaction to its strength and effects.

1 (14-ounce) can coconut milk
1 cup water
1 tablespoon canna-oil (page 105)
2 teaspoons ground turmeric
¼ teaspoon ground cinnamon
1 tablespoon honey
¼ teaspoon freshly grated or ground ginger
Pinch cayenne pepper (optional)
Pinch freshly ground black pepper

1. In a small saucepan, combine all the ingredients. Heat over medium-low heat for 5 minutes until hot. Remove from the heat.

2. Using an immersion blender, blend on low speed until smooth.

3. Pour into mugs and serve immediately.

- -

To reduce the calories and fat in this recipe, replace the coconut milk with an equal amount of almond milk. You can use 1 tablespoon of canna-butter or 1½ teaspoons of cannabis tincture in place of the canna-oil.

PER SERVING Calories: 373; Total Fat: 36.2g; Saturated Fat: 32g; Cholesterol: 0mg; Carbohydrates: 14.9g; Fiber: 37g; Protein: 3.2g

FRESH-PRESSED CANNA-JUICE

GLUTEN-FREE | NUT-FREE | SOY-FREE | SUGAR-FREE | VEGAN

For a fresh drink without the psychotropic effects of THC, raw cannabis juice is the way to go. Fresh cannabis is loaded with the cannabinoid THCA and a bouquet of terpenes that are often burned away when smoking or vaping. Ingesting cannabis raw is the surest way to get all those wonderful medicinal benefits.

MAKES 24 OUNCES

[8 ounces = 1 serving]
Prep time: 10 minutes, plus
   overnight soaking

Required Equipment
Blender
Cheesecloth
Fine mesh strainer

 DOSAGE TEST

Start with half of a serving of canna-juice and wait 4 hours to fully assess your reaction to its strength and effects.

20 raw cannabis leaves
4 cups water

1. Rinse the cannabis leaves.

2. In a large bowl, combine the cannabis and water. Cover and soak overnight.

3. Transfer both the soaking water and leaves to a blender. Blend for 1 to 2 minutes until liquefied.

4. Line a fine mesh strainer with cheesecloth and place it over a large bowl. Carefully pour the juice through the cheesecloth. Press to extract any remaining liquid through the cheesecloth.

5. Transfer to glass jars, and store in the refrigerator for up to 3 days or in the freezer in a freezer-safe container for up to 6 months.

For a flavor boost, replace the water with an equal amount of coconut water and add 2 tablespoons of fresh lime juice and 2 tablespoons of honey.

CANNABIS TINCTURE

GLUTEN-FREE | NUT-FREE | SOY-FREE | VEGAN

Tinctures can be administered under the tongue for quick delivery. Unlike edibles, effects are usually felt within minutes. While many tinctures are alcohol-based, we prefer the taste and gentleness of tinctures with a vegetable glycerin base, and you may find that the same is true for you.

MAKES 12 OUNCES

[½ teaspoon = 1 serving]
Prep time: 5 minutes
Cook time: 45 minutes
Infusion time: 2 months

Required Equipment
Cheesecloth

 DOSAGE TEST

Start with ⅛ teaspoon (12 drops) of cannabis tincture under the tongue and wait 4 hours to fully assess your reaction to its strength and effects.

14 grams cannabis, coarsely ground
12 ounces vegetable glycerin

1. Preheat the oven to 240ºF.

2. Place the cannabis on a rimmed baking sheet and bake for 45 minutes to activate the THC, resulting in decarboxylated cannabis.

3. Transfer the decarboxylated cannabis to a glass jar.

4. Pour the glycerin over the cannabis, being sure that the glycerin covers the cannabis completely.

5. Secure the jar with an airtight lid and gently stir the contents by rolling the jar back and forth in your hands.

6. Keep the jar in a dark place at room temperature for 2 months. Agitate the contents of the jar intermittently (once or twice a week is fine) by rolling it back and forth in your hands.

7. Stretch cheesecloth across the top of a large, spouted measuring cup or bowl, and secure with a rubber band or twine around the edge.

8. Carefully pour the infused glycerin over the cheesecloth.

➤

CANNABIS TINCTURE

CONTINUED

9. Lift the cheesecloth and squeeze any remaining glycerin into the measuring cup or bowl.

10. Pour the tincture back into the glass jar or dropper bottles. Store in a cool, dark place or in the refrigerator for up to 18 months.

- -

To use, place a few drops under the tongue and allow it to absorb before swallowing. If you find the taste displeasing, you can add it to a sweet beverage. ■ *In our kitchen, we cook with cannabis that has 15 percent THC, which results in 10 milligrams of THC per ½ teaspoon of this tincture. If you need a higher or lower dose, you can use more or less cannabis when making your tincture.*

PER SERVING Calories: 11; Total Fat: 0g; Saturated Fat: 0g; Cholesterol: 0mg; Carbohydrates: 2.5g; Fiber: 0g; Protein: 0g

CANNA-HONEY

GLUTEN-FREE | NUT-FREE | SOY-FREE | VEGETARIAN

Like cannabis, honey has anti-inflammatory, antibacterial, and healing properties. It can also reduce nausea, alleviate allergy symptoms, boost memory, and suppress coughs. This recipe calls for cannabis tincture because straight cannabis alone does not infuse efficiently with honey.

MAKES 12 OUNCES
[1 tablespoon = 1 serving]
Prep time: 5 minutes

 DOSAGE TEST

Start with 1 teaspoon of canna-honey and wait 4 hours to fully assess your reaction to its strength and effects.

10 ounces honey
2 ounces cannabis tincture (page 119)

1. In a small saucepan, warm the honey over low heat until thin.

2. Remove from the heat, and add the tincture. Stir well.

3. Pour into a glass jar or honey jar and store in your pantry as you would regular honey.

- -

In our kitchen, we cook with cannabis that has 15 percent THC, which results in 10 milligrams of THC per tablespoon of this honey. If you need a higher or lower dose, you can use more or less tincture when making this honey.

PER SERVING Calories: 64; Total Fat: 0g; Saturated Fat: 0g; Cholesterol: 0mg; Carbohydrates: 17g; Fiber: 0g; Protein: 0.1g

CANNABIS LOZENGES

GLUTEN-FREE | NUT-FREE | SOY-FREE | VEGETARIAN

Lozenges and other hard candies infused with cannabis can have a faster onset than traditional chew-and-swallow edibles. The cannabinoids are absorbed in the mouth and sent to the brain more quickly than when digested in the stomach and processed in the liver. But, just as the onset may be faster, the duration may also be shorter.

MAKES 18 LOZENGES

[1 lozenge = 1 serving]
Prep time: 10 minutes
Cook time: 15 minutes

Required Equipment
Candy thermometer
Candy molds

 DOSAGE TEST

Start with one-half of a lozenge and wait 4 hours to fully assess your reaction to its strength and effects.

½ cup honey
2 tablespoons apple cider vinegar
2 tablespoons freshly grated ginger
½ teaspoon ground cinnamon
1½ tablespoons cannabis tincture (page 119)
⅓ cup powdered sugar

1. In a heavy saucepan, combine the honey, vinegar, ginger, and cinnamon. Bring to a boil over medium heat.

2. Insert the candy thermometer and continue to boil until the thermometer reaches 300ºF.

3. Remove from the heat and quickly stir in the tincture, mixing vigorously for even distribution.

4. Carefully pour the hot mixture into the candy molds. Allow them to cool and harden.

5. Remove the lozenges from the molds and toss with powdered sugar.

6. Store in an airtight container in the refrigerator for up to 3 months.

- -

If you don't have candy molds, line 2 rimmed baking sheets with parchment paper. Allow the mixture to cool slightly, then carefully pour the mixture into small circles. If it spreads too much, allow the mixture to cool a bit longer. For a fruity lozenge, omit the ginger and cinnamon and add a flavored extract along with the tincture. ■ In our kitchen, we cook with cannabis that has 15 percent THC, which results in 5 milligrams of THC per lozenge. If you need a higher or lower dose, you can increase or decrease the amount of tincture in this recipe.

PER SERVING Calories: 31; Total Fat: 0g; Saturated Fat: 0g; Cholesterol: 0mg; Carbohydrates: 8.2g; Fiber: 0g; Protein: 0.1g

CANNABIS COUGH SYRUP

GLUTEN-FREE | NUT-FREE | SOY-FREE | VEGETARIAN

Honey and ginger pair up again in this effective cough syrup. Pepper and thyme are unexpected additions to this remedy, but they each have potent properties that fight cough and congestion.

MAKES 6 OUNCES

[1 tablespoon = 1 serving]
Prep time: 10 minutes
Cook time: 5 minutes

 DOSAGE TEST

Start with 1 teaspoon of cough syrup and wait 4 hours to fully assess your reaction to its strength and effects.

½ cup honey
3 tablespoons freshly squeezed lemon juice
3 tablespoons cannabis tincture (page 119)
2 teaspoons freshly grated or ground ginger
1 teaspoon white pepper
1 teaspoon ground thyme

1. In a small saucepan, combine the honey, lemon juice, and tincture. Heat over low heat for 1 to 2 minutes until the honey thins.

2. Add the ginger, pepper, and thyme, and stir. Continue to warm over low heat for 3 to 4 minutes. Remove from the heat.

3. Allow the syrup to cool slightly before transferring to an airtight container. Store in the refrigerator for up to 3 weeks.

- -

In our kitchen, we cook with cannabis that has 15 percent THC, which results in 10 milligrams of THC per tablespoon of this cough syrup. If you need a higher or lower dose, you can increase or decrease the amount of tincture in this recipe.

PER SERVING Calories: 46; Total Fat: 0g; Saturated Fat: 0g; Cholesterol: 0mg; Carbohydrates: 12g; Fiber: 0g; Protein: 0g

CANNABIS SUPPOSITORY

GLUTEN-FREE | NUT-FREE | SOY-FREE

Suppositories offer an efficient uptake of cannabis if you cannot or do not wish to inhale or ingest cannabis. This can be an important delivery method if you have extreme nausea and vomiting. It has also been shown to be a helpful remedy for gastro-intestinal issues.

MAKES 60 SUPPOSITORIES

Prep time: 5 minutes
Cook time: 2 minutes

Required Equipment

60 (2.3-milliliter) suppository molds

 DOSAGE TEST

Start with 1 suppository and wait 4 hours to fully assess your reaction to its strength and effects. Remaining suppositories can be melted if too strong or too weak. Start over with a new batch of canna-oil, adjusting the ratio of cannabis to oil as necessary.

6 tablespoons canna-oil (page 105)

1. In a small saucepan, melt the canna-oil over low heat.

2. Pour the warm oil into the suppository molds.

3. Place the molds in the refrigerator to solidify.

4. Store in the refrigerator for up to 1 year.

- -

In our kitchen, we cook with cannabis that has 15 percent THC, which results in 3 milligrams of THC per cannabis suppository. If you need a higher or lower dose, increase or decrease the amount of cannabis in the canna-oil recipe.

Essential Oil Blends

The recipes that follow can be made with essential oils, which have long been used in herbal remedies. Because some people may have adverse reactions due to skin sensitivities and allergies, it's important to test new essential oils before using them. To do so, dilute the essential oil (add one drop of it to one teaspoon of a carrier oil, such as almond oil or coconut oil) and apply a small amount to the inside of your elbow or wrist. Wait 24 hours to assess your skin's reaction. Do not wash the test patch during those 24 hours. If your skin does not show signs of swelling, redness, or itching, you can consider the essential oil safe to use.

FOR SALVES AND LOTIONS

For All-Purpose Pain Relief: 4 drops camphor; 3 drops peppermint; 2 drops eucalyptus; 1 drop cloves; 2 drops cinnamon

For All-Purpose Soothing Relief: 5 drops lavender; 4 drops lemon; 3 drops melaleuca

For Muscle and Joint Pain, Arthritis, Fibromyalgia: 4 drops birch; 4 drops geranium; 4 drops lemongrass

For Headaches and Migraines: 6 drops lavender; 4 drops lemongrass; 2 drops peppermint

FOR SOAKS

For Arthritis: 8 drops juniper; 4 drops lavender; 4 drops cypress; 4 drops rosemary

For Headaches and Migraines: 13 drops lavender; 7 drops chamomile

For Muscle Pain and Fibromyalgia: 5 drops eucalyptus; 5 drops rosemary; 5 drops lavender; 5 drops cinnamon

FOR STEAMS

For Congestion and Inflamed Sinuses: Eucalyptus or pine

For Cold and Cough: Rosemary

For Relaxation: Lavender or chamomile

CANNABIS SALVE

Cannabis salve provides localized pain relief without THC's psychoactive effects. When applied to the skin, this salve can soothe sore muscles, joints, arthritis, nerve pain, headaches, migraines, and cramps. This remedy can be personalized with the essential oil blend that suits your needs.

MAKES 8 OUNCES
Prep time: 20 minutes

 DOSAGE TEST

Apply salve to a small area of your skin and wait 4 hours to fully assess your reaction to its strength and effects.

½ cup canna-oil (page 105)
½ cup hemp seed oil
2 tablespoons grated beeswax
½ teaspoon vitamin E oil
12 drops essential oil blend (page 125)

1. In a 1-pint mason jar, combine the canna-oil, hemp seed oil, and beeswax.

2. Fill a large saucepan halfway with water. Place the uncovered mason jar in the saucepan, ensuring that no water gets into the jar.

3. Heat over medium-low heat, stirring occasionally, until all the beeswax has melted.

4. Remove from the heat and add the vitamin E oil and essential oil blend. Stir until thoroughly incorporated.

5. Carefully pour the mixture into two 4-ounce jars. Allow to cool completely before sealing with an airtight lid.

6. Store at room temperature for up to 1 year.

- -

If the consistency is too hard upon cooling, transfer to the larger jar, repeat steps 2 and 3, and add a little extra hemp seed oil. If the consistency is too soft upon cooling, transfer to the larger jar and repeat steps 2 and 3 with a little extra beeswax.

CANNABIS BODY LOTION

This wonderfully creamy lotion is a breeze to whip up. Like the cannabis salve, this lotion is a great localized pain treatment without the psychotropic effects of THC. Cannabis has also been shown to effectively treat psoriasis.

MAKES 2 CUPS

Prep time: 15 minutes

Required Equipment
Blender

 DOSAGE TEST

Apply lotion to a small area of your skin and wait 4 hours to fully assess your reaction to its strength and effects.

¾ cup canna-oil (page 105)
3 tablespoons grated beeswax
1 teaspoon vitamin E oil (optional)
1 cup filtered water

1. In a 1-pint mason jar, combine the canna-oil and beeswax.

2. Fill a large saucepan halfway with water. Place the uncovered mason jar in the saucepan, ensuring that no water gets into the jar.

3. Heat over low to medium heat, stirring occasionally, until all the beeswax has melted.

4. Remove from the heat and add the vitamin E oil (if using). Stir until thoroughly incorporated.

5. Pour the water into a blender and begin blending at medium speed. Remove the blender cap and slowly pour in the oil-wax mixture while continuing to blend.

6. Replace the blender cap, and continue to blend for 1 to 2 minutes until the water and the wax-oil mixture have emulsified.

7. Transfer to clean jars and allow to cool completely before covering with an airtight lid. Store in the refrigerator for up to 3 months.

- -

For a fragrant twist, you can replace the water in this recipe with an equal amount of cold brewed tea, rosewater, or orange blossom water. You can also add up to 10 drops of essential oil (page 125) when you add the vitamin E.

CANNABIS BATH SOAK

Salt bath soaks and cannabis are both known to help psoriasis, arthritis, fibromyalgia, joint pain, and muscle pain. Put them together, and you've got a double-powered treatment. Dead Sea salt is high in magnesium, potassium, and calcium chlorides, and baking soda helps detoxify and soften the skin. This bath soak can be personalized with the essential oil blend that suits your needs.

MAKES 4 CUPS

[1 cup per bath]
Prep time: 10 minutes

 DOSAGE TEST

Start with ¼ cup of cannabis bath soak and wait 4 hours to fully assess your reaction to its strength and effects.

2 tablespoons canna-oil (page 105)
20 drops essential oil blend (page 125)
2 cups Dead Sea salt
1 cup Epsom salt
1 cup baking soda

1. In a small saucepan, soften the canna-oil over low heat until just melted. Remove from the heat.

2. Add the essential oil blend to the melted oil, and stir until thoroughly incorporated.

3. In a medium mixing bowl, combine the oil mixture, salts, and baking soda. Stir until evenly combined.

4. Transfer to glass jars. Store in a cool, dark place for up to 6 months.

- -

As long as you don't swallow your bathwater (and, please, do not swallow your bathwater), this treatment is nonpsychoactive. Keep the water warm, but not too hot; below 104°F is ideal. If you have diabetes, omit the Epsom salt, which can trigger the release of insulin. ■ *You can replace the canna-oil with cannabis tincture if you prefer.*

CANNABIS STEAM BOWL

An age-old remedy for nasal and upper-respiratory relief, steam bowls are an effective way to treat congestion and infections and a novel way to deliver your cannabis. In this treatment, cannabis tincture or canna-oil is added to hot, steaming water along with essential oils to treat your respiratory issues.

MAKES 1 TREATMENT
Prep time: 10 minutes

 DOSAGE TEST

Start with 1 teaspoon of canna-oil (or ½ teaspoon of tincture) in your steam bowl and wait 4 hours to fully assess your reaction to its strength and effects.

1 tablespoon canna-oil (page 105) or
   1½ teaspoons cannabis tincture (page 119)
4 drops essential oil (page 125)
4 to 6 cups water

1. In a large bowl, combine the canna-oil or cannabis tincture and the essential oil.

2. In a medium pot, heat the water until it is hot but not boiling.

3. Pour the hot water into the bowl and allow the water to cool until the steam is warm.

4. Place a towel over your head, and lower your face until you're about 8 to 12 inches from the bowl. Keep your eyes closed. Breathe deeply until the water has stopped steaming.

- -

You can omit the essential oils if you are sensitive to scents, or use an essential oil that isn't listed if you have a different preference. ■ *Steam twice a day until respiratory relief is achieved.*

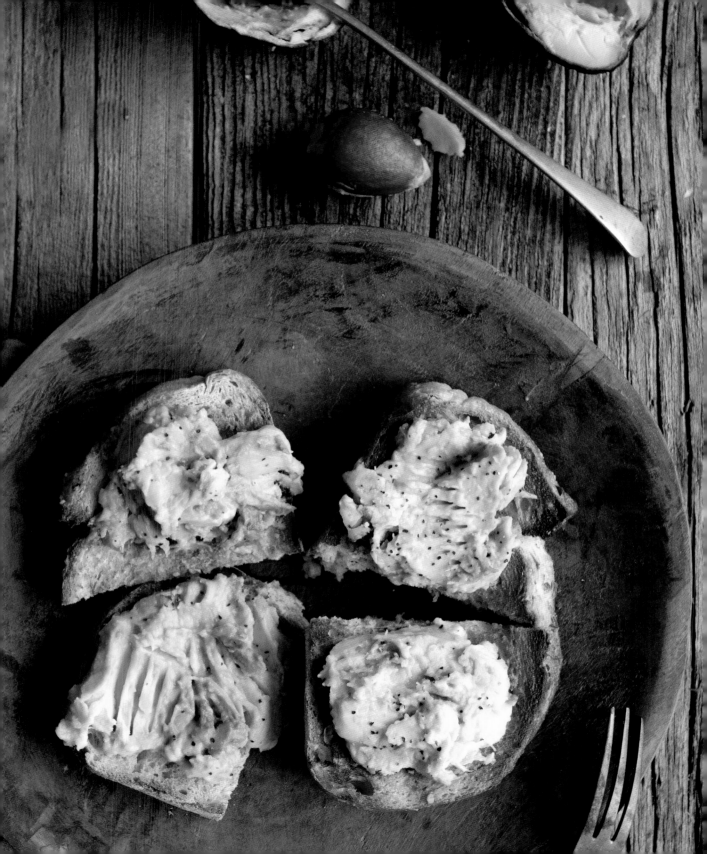

SAVORY CANNABIS EDIBLES

WITH CANNA-BUTTER (page 106) or canna-oil (page 105) on hand, you can prepare the majority of these savory recipes quickly. When you make your own edibles, you can be sure of the dosage and integrity of all the ingredients. And, most important, you can tailor them to meet your dietary and health needs. All of these recipes are simple and healthy, and use ingredients (aside from the cannabis-infused oil and butter) that can easily be found at your local grocery store. Bon appétit!

Required Equipment

Most of the recipes in this chapter don't require any equipment other than a stove top, oven, and pots and pans. Aside from these basic kitchen tools, a couple of the recipes call for the following items.

Blender—This kitchen appliance is used to blend, purée, and liquefy. You can use a standard blender or an immersion blender. You can find a blender online or at your local kitchen and home supply store.

Food Processor—This versatile machine is used for slicing, shredding, grinding, puréeing, and blending. You can find a food processor online or at your local kitchen and home supply store.

Waxed Paper Bags—Waxed paper bags (such as the ones in which baked goods are stored) make it easy to cook in the microwave while retaining the flavor and moistness of the edible contents. They can be found online and in most grocery stores.

THOUGHTS AND EXPERIENCES

M y mother, who is 87 and diabetic, was in incredible pain and had no appetite. Before treating her with cannabis, my brothers and I felt helpless. We would take her to the doctor only to be told to keep doing what we were doing, but she was slowly wasting away. She had no energy. After using medical marijuana, her condition improved. This is what she has to say:

"I love marijuana. I wish I had understood it earlier. When all the kids were doing it, I thought they would get hooked. None of you did, obviously. The pills I was taking before made it so I couldn't go to the bathroom on my own. Now I can. And I can sit in a normal chair. I got my appetite back. I was getting too skinny. It's those soups you all make for me with that oil. And the doctor can't believe it. He has been my doctor for 20 years. I keep asking him to try it, but you know how doctors are."

Watching my mother's transformation has been amazing. She has really gotten her strength back. I was nervous about giving her cannabis oil at first, but we talked with her about the new medical research, and she agreed. We all had a good laugh about the idea of Mom on marijuana. We usually put a small amount of the oil in soup or oatmeal for her, once or maybe twice a day. She tells us it eases her pain, and we've all seen her appetite come back in full force! She asks us to bring treats when we come over now. It is wonderful to see her enjoying life again. —**Carol C.**, Washington

EGG NOODLES
WITH COTTAGE CHEESE

NUT-FREE | SOY-FREE | SUGAR-FREE | VEGETARIAN

This noodle dish is good anytime, but it is especially comforting if you're feeling under the weather. There is something simple and pure about it—and it's so easy to prepare.

MAKES 2 SERVINGS

Prep time: 5 minutes
Cook time: 15 minutes

 DOSAGE TEST

Start with half of a serving and wait 4 hours to fully assess your reaction to its strength and effects.

8 ounces egg noodles
1 tablespoon butter
2 teaspoons canna-butter (page 106)
1 cup cottage cheese, at room temperature
Salt
Freshly ground black pepper

1. Cook the noodles according to the package directions. Drain the noodles and transfer to a large bowl.

2. Add the butters, and stir until melted.

3. Add the cottage cheese, and stir to combine. Season with salt and pepper.

4. Serve warm.

5. Store the remaining serving in an airtight container in the refrigerator for up to 4 days. Reheat in the microwave on low power for 2 minutes or until warm.

- -

To bring the cottage cheese to room temperature, let it sit on the countertop for one hour. If you use it straight from the refrigerator, you'll be left with cold noodles.

PER SERVING Calories: 270; Total Fat: 9.7g; Saturated Fat: 5.4g; Cholesterol: 49mg; Carbohydrates: 25.5g; Fiber: 1g; Protein: 19.5g

QUINOA
WITH MIXED VEGETABLES

NUT-FREE | SOY-FREE | SUGAR-FREE | VEGAN

Quinoa is a luscious, filling grain. This dish makes a perfect one-bowl meal for breakfast, lunch, or dinner.

MAKES 2 SERVINGS
Prep time: 5 minutes
Cook time: 20 minutes

 DOSAGE TEST

Start with half of a serving and wait 4 hours to fully assess your reaction to its strength and effects.

2¾ cups vegetable broth
1½ cups quinoa
1 (16-ounce) package frozen mixed vegetables (any type)
1 tablespoon olive oil
2 teaspoons canna-oil (page 105)
Salt
Freshly ground black pepper

1. In a medium saucepan, combine the broth and quinoa. Bring to a boil.

2. Add the vegetables, reduce the heat, and cover. Simmer for 12 to 15 minutes until the liquid is absorbed. Remove from the heat and allow to sit for 5 minutes.

3. Transfer to a medium bowl and add the oils. Stir to combine. Season with salt and pepper.

4. Serve warm.

5. Store the remaining serving in an airtight container in the refrigerator for up to 3 days. Reheat in the microwave on low power for 2 minutes or until warm.

- -

For a super-healthy alternative to fried rice, stir-fry your leftovers with a beaten egg in a hot pan with a light coating of canola oil.

PER SERVING Calories: 291; Total Fat: 8.3g; Saturated Fat: 1.2g; Cholesterol: 0mg; Carbohydrates: 41.6g; Fiber: 4.5g; Protein: 12.3g

SUPER GRILLED CHEESE

NUT-FREE | SOY-FREE | SUGAR-FREE | VEGETARIAN

Grilled cheese with cannabis might be the world's ultimate comfort food. This recipe calls for Cheddar and Swiss, but you can swap them out for other types of cheese. With the addition of one or more of the optional items, you can customize this sandwich to suit your taste.

MAKES 2 SERVINGS

Prep time: 10 minutes
Cook time: 10 minutes

 DOSAGE TEST

Start with half of a serving and wait 4 hours to fully assess your reaction to its strength and effects.

4 slices whole-wheat or whole-grain bread
2 teaspoons canna-butter (page 106), at room temperature
4 slices Cheddar cheese
4 slices Swiss cheese
2 slices tomato, avocado, and/or grilled vegetables (optional)
1 tablespoon olive oil

1. Butter 2 bread slices with the canna-butter.

2. On the buttered side of each bread slice, place 2 slices of the Cheddar cheese and 2 slices of the Swiss cheese.

3. Add the tomato, avocado, and/or grilled vegetables (if using).

4. Close the sandwiches with the other 2 bread slices.

5. In a large, nonstick skillet, heat the olive oil, allowing it to spread around the pan. Place the sandwiches in the skillet and cook over medium heat for 5 to 6 minutes until golden brown. Flip the sandwiches and cook for 4 to 5 minutes until golden brown.

6. Serve warm.

7. Store the remaining serving in an airtight container in the refrigerator for up to 1 week. Reheat in a skillet over medium heat for a few minutes on each side until hot. (Do not use avocado if you plan to store it.)

- -

For a flavor boost, spread 1 to 2 teaspoons of mustard on the bread before closing the sandwiches. Other optional sandwich fillings include apple slices or even pickle slices.

PER SERVING Calories: 522; Total Fat: 35.3g; Saturated Fat: 18.3g; Cholesterol: 85mg; Carbohydrates: 27.2g; Fiber: 4g; Protein: 27.5g

HUMMUS

GLUTEN-FREE | NUT-FREE | SOY-FREE | SUGAR-FREE | VEGAN

Hummus is simple and nourishing. Serve it alongside vegetables or chips as a dip or use it as a spread. Or, add cucumber slices to make a delicious and oh-so-soothing sandwich.

MAKES 1½ CUPS

[6 tablespoons = 1 serving]
Prep time: 10 minutes

Required Equipment
Food processor

 DOSAGE TEST

Start with half of a serving and wait 4 hours to fully assess your reaction to its strength and effects.

1 (15-ounce) can chickpeas, rinsed and drained
1 garlic clove
¼ cup olive oil
4 teaspoons canna-oil (page 105)
2 tablespoons freshly squeezed lemon juice
2 teaspoons ground cumin
½ teaspoon ground paprika
½ teaspoon ground turmeric
Pinch salt

1. Combine all the ingredients in a food processor.

2. Pulse a few times, and then purée for 1 to 2 minutes until smooth.

3. Transfer from the food processor to a serving dish.

4. Serve at room temperature.

5. Store the remaining servings in the refrigerator in an airtight container for up to 2 weeks.

- -

When making this hummus, you can blend in the flesh of a cooked sweet potato, ¼ cup roasted red pepper, or even a handful of fresh spinach.

PER SERVING Calories: 243; Total Fat: 14.2g; Saturated Fat: 2g; Cholesterol: 0mg; Carbohydrates: 25.2g; Fiber: 5g; Protein: 5.6g

CARROT-GINGER SOUP

GLUTEN-FREE | NUT-FREE | SOY-FREE | SUGAR-FREE | VEGAN

Carrots and ginger are a flavorful combination. The ginger in this recipe perfectly complements the sweet carrots.

MAKES 2 SERVINGS

Prep time: 10 minutes
Cook time: 40 minutes

Required Equipment
Blender

 DOSAGE TEST

Start with half of a serving and wait 4 hours to fully assess your reaction to its strength and effects.

1 tablespoon olive oil
2 teaspoons canna-oil (page 105)
1 small onion, peeled and chopped
2 garlic cloves, minced
1 teaspoon grated fresh ginger or ½ teaspoon ground ginger
1 pound carrots, scrubbed and chopped
2 cups vegetable stock

1. In a medium saucepan, combine the oils and heat over low heat. Add the onion and garlic, and sauté for 7 to 10 minutes.

2. Add the ginger and the carrots, and sauté for an additional 4 to 5 minutes.

3. Add the vegetable stock, and simmer for 20 to 25 minutes until the carrots are tender.

4. Allow the soup to cool and transfer to a blender. Purée for 1 to 2 minutes until smooth.

5. Reheat the soup over medium heat until hot.

6. Serve warm.

7. Store the remaining serving in an airtight container in the refrigerator for up to 1 week. Reheat in a small saucepan over low heat.

- -

If you prefer chicken broth, you can use it in place of the vegetable broth; it's an even swap.

PER SERVING Calories: 117; Total Fat: 0.2g; Saturated Fat: 0g; Cholesterol: 0mg; Carbohydrates: 27.5g; Fiber: 6.9g; Protein: 2.8g

DOUBLE-STRENGTH
CHICKEN SOUP
WITH TOMATO TOAST

NUT-FREE | SOY-FREE | SUGAR-FREE

Dill is called for in this tasty soup, but you can use parsley or cilantro in its place to suit your preference. If you have cooked chicken on hand, you can add it to the chicken stock and cut down on the cooking time.

MAKES 4 SERVINGS

Prep time: 10 minutes
Cook time: 1 hour, 30 minutes

 DOSAGE TEST

Start with half of a serving and wait 4 hours to fully assess your reaction to its strength and effects.

1 quart chicken stock
4 bone-in, skinless chicken thighs
2 teaspoons canna-oil (page 105)
2 carrots, peeled and sliced
1 celery stalk, sliced
1 tablespoon chopped fresh dill
4 baguette slices
1 tomato, halved

1. In a medium soup pot, heat the chicken stock over medium heat. Add the chicken thighs and cook for 20 minutes, skimming off the foam that rises to the top.

2. Add the canna-oil, carrots, celery, and dill. Continue to cook for 1 hour. Remove from the heat.

3. Using tongs, remove the chicken from the pot, and transfer to a cutting board. Remove the meat from the bones and chop roughly. Return the meat to the pot.

4. Toast the baguette slices. Rub the cut sides of the tomato generously on each toasted slice.

5. Divide the soup into 2 bowls, and serve the toast on the side. Serve warm.

6. Store the remaining serving in an airtight container in the refrigerator for up to 3 days. Reheat in a small saucepan over low heat. (Toast the baguette slices separately.)

- -

For a more traditional soup, add 2 cups of cooked egg noodles.

PER SERVING Calories: 120; Total Fat: 1.2g; Saturated Fat: 0g; Cholesterol: 0mg; Carbohydrates: 23g; Fiber: 1.9g; Protein: 5g

CABBAGE SOUP

GLUTEN-FREE | NUT-FREE | SOY-FREE | SUGAR-FREE

This humble soup is almost like a hearty veggie stew. The flavorful broth will take you by surprise, and it's even better the day after you make it.

MAKES 6 SERVINGS

Prep time: 10 minutes
Cook time: 45 minutes

 DOSAGE TEST

Start with half of a serving and wait 4 hours to fully assess your reaction to its strength and effects.

2 tablespoons canna-oil (page 105)
8 ounces lean ground beef or ground turkey
1 bell pepper, seeded and chopped
1 cup sliced, peeled carrots
½ cup chopped onion
3 garlic cloves, minced
3 cups coarsely chopped green cabbage
6 cups water
1 (15-ounce) can diced fire-roasted tomatoes
1 teaspoon smoked paprika
¼ teaspoon salt
Freshly ground black pepper

1. Heat the canna-oil in a large soup pot over medium heat. Add the ground meat and sauté for 6 to 7 minutes. Drain off the fat.

2. Add the bell pepper, carrots, onion, and garlic, and sauté for 10 to 12 minutes until tender.

3. Add the cabbage and sauté briefly until wilted.

4. Add the water, tomatoes with their juice, paprika, salt, and pepper, and simmer for 25 to 30 minutes.

5. Serve warm.

6. Store the remaining servings in an airtight container in the refrigerator for up to 1 week. Reheat in a small saucepan over low heat.

- -

To add a bit of spice to your soup, when sautéing the beef or turkey, add 4 ounces of hot Italian sausage removed from its casing.

PER SERVING Calories: 77; Total Fat: 2.4g; Saturated Fat: 0.9g; Cholesterol: 34mg; Carbohydrates: 1.6g; Fiber: 0g; Protein: 11.7g

ASPARAGUS SOUP

GLUTEN-FREE | NUT-FREE | SOY-FREE | SUGAR-FREE | VEGETARIAN

This cold soup is wonderfully refreshing on a summer day. However, it is equally delicious served hot. Simply return the soup to the pot after puréeing and heat.

MAKES 6 SERVINGS

Prep time: 10 minutes
Cook time: 20 minutes, plus
  3 hours chilling time

Required Equipment
Blender

 DOSAGE TEST

Start with half of a serving and wait 4 hours to fully assess your reaction to its strength and effects.

2 tablespoons canna-butter (page 106)
2 leeks, white and light green parts only, roughly chopped
2 pounds asparagus, trimmed and roughly chopped
4 cups vegetable stock
Pinch salt
Freshly ground black pepper
6 tablespoons Greek yogurt, for garnish
Finely chopped chives, for garnish

1. In a large soup pot, melt the canna-butter over low heat. Add the leeks, and sauté over medium heat for 7 to 10 minutes until soft.

2. Add the asparagus and vegetable stock. Bring to a boil over high heat.

3. Reduce the heat, cover, and simmer for 8 to 10 minutes until the asparagus is tender.

4. Allow the soup to cool and transfer to a blender. Purée for about 1 minute until smooth.

5. Transfer the puréed soup to a large bowl and season with salt and pepper.

6. Allow the mixture to chill in the refrigerator for at least 3 hours.

7. Serve in a chilled bowl with a dollop of yogurt and garnish with chives.

8. Store the remaining servings in an airtight container in the refrigerator for up to 5 days. (Add the yogurt and garnish only when ready to eat.)

- -

This soup can be made with zucchini instead of asparagus. With zucchini, garnish with fresh dill instead of chives.

PER SERVING Calories: 48; Total Fat: 0.3g; Saturated Fat: 0g; Cholesterol: 0mg; Carbohydrates: 10.1g; Fiber: 3.7g; Protein: 3.8g

THAI CHICKEN SOUP

GLUTEN-FREE | NUT-FREE | SOY-FREE

If you have never tried this soup in a Thai restaurant, you don't know how yummy it is. It is easy to make at home, and although some of the ingredients may be new to you, the flavors work together beautifully.

MAKES 2 SERVINGS

Prep time: 10 minutes
Cook time: 30 minutes

 DOSAGE TEST

Start with half of a serving and wait 4 hours to fully assess your reaction to its strength and effects.

2 teaspoons canna-oil (page 105)
½ cup sliced white mushrooms
½ bell pepper, chopped
1 garlic clove, minced
2 cups canned chicken broth
1 cup canned coconut milk
2 teaspoons fish sauce
2 teaspoons honey
1 cup sliced or chopped cooked chicken
1 scallion, chopped, for garnish

1. In a medium saucepan, heat the canna-oil over medium heat. Add the mushrooms, bell pepper, and garlic and sauté for 5 to 7 minutes.

2. Add the broth, coconut milk, fish sauce, honey, and chicken, and simmer for 25 minutes.

3. Serve warm, garnished with the scallion.

4. Store the remaining serving in an airtight container in the refrigerator for up to 3 days. Reheat in a small saucepan over low heat.

- -

If you are not a fan of fish sauce, you can simply eliminate it from the recipe. This soup is also terrific with shrimp (precooked or added during the last 10 minutes of cooking time) in place of the chicken.

PER SERVING Calories: 325; Total Fat: 30.1g; Saturated Fat: 25.8g; Cholesterol: 0mg; Carbohydrates: 17g; Fiber: 3.7g; Protein: 9g

RICE AND BEAN BOWL

GLUTEN-FREE | NUT-FREE | SOY-FREE | SUGAR-FREE | VEGAN

Rice and beans is an excellent side dish, or with a few additions, it can be a complete meal. This recipe welcomes a generous portion of tofu or cooked chicken for a more protein-rich dish.

MAKES 4 SERVINGS

Prep time: 10 minutes
Cook time: 20 minutes

 DOSAGE TEST

Start with half of a serving and wait 4 hours to fully assess your reaction to its strength and effects.

4 teaspoons canna-oil (page 105)
1 onion, peeled and chopped
1 cup vegetable broth
1 (16-ounce) can kidney beans, rinsed and drained
1 (10-ounce) package frozen spinach, thawed and squeezed of liquid
2 cups cooked brown or white rice
Salt
Freshly ground black pepper

1. In a large sauté pan or skillet, heat the canna-oil over medium heat. Add the onion, and sauté for 5 to 7 minutes.

2. Add the broth, beans, and spinach, and simmer for 5 minutes.

3. Add the cooked rice, and simmer for 5 to 7 minutes. Season with salt and pepper.

4. Serve warm.

5. Store the remaining servings in an airtight container in the refrigerator for up to 5 days. Reheat in the microwave on low power for 2 minutes or until warm.

- -

Use leftovers as a burrito filling with a dollop of sour cream and a few tablespoons of salsa.

PER SERVING Calories: 331; Total Fat: 7.7g; Saturated Fat: 1.2g; Cholesterol: 0mg; Carbohydrates: 111.2g; Fiber: 21.2g; Protein: 32.7g

KALE, CHICKPEA, AND CAULIFLOWER SOUP

GLUTEN-FREE | NUT-FREE | SOY-FREE | SUGAR-FREE | VEGAN

This is a perfect soup for a blustery day. It is quite chunky, so if you prefer a smoother soup, purée a few cups in the blender and add them back to the pot.

MAKES 4 SERVINGS

Prep time: 10 minutes
Cook time: 50 minutes

 DOSAGE TEST

Start with half of a serving and wait 4 hours to fully assess your reaction to its strength and effects.

4 teaspoons canna-oil (page 105)
1 head cauliflower, broken into florets
½ cup shredded carrot
1 garlic clove, minced
1 (15-ounce) can chickpeas, rinsed and drained
2 cups shredded kale leaves
5 cups vegetable broth
Salt
Freshly ground black pepper

1. In a large saucepot, heat the canna-oil over medium heat. Add the cauliflower, carrot, and garlic, and sauté for 8 to 10 minutes.

2. Add the chickpeas and kale, and sauté for 5 minutes.

3. Add the broth and simmer for 35 to 40 minutes, stirring occasionally. Season with salt and pepper.

4. Serve warm.

5. Store the remaining servings in an airtight container in the refrigerator for up to 4 days. Reheat in a small saucepan over low heat.

- -

If you are not a chickpea fan, you can use a different type of legume.

PER SERVING Calories: 240; Total Fat: 3g; Saturated Fat: 0.6g; Cholesterol: 0mg; Carbohydrates: 33.8g; Fiber: 7.2g; Protein: 13.8g

AVOCADO TOAST

NUT-FREE | SOY-FREE | SUGAR-FREE | VEGETARIAN

This recipe begs for a ripe, beautiful avocado. Pick one that yields to gentle pressure. Avocado browns easily when cut, so drizzle it with lemon juice after peeling to keep it looking fresh.

MAKES 2 SERVINGS

Prep time: 10 minutes

 DOSAGE TEST

Start with half of a serving and wait 4 hours to fully assess your reaction to its strength and effects.

2 slices whole-grain bread
2 teaspoons canna-butter (page 106), at room temperature
4 slices ripe tomato (optional)
1 large avocado, peeled, pitted, and sliced
2 teaspoons freshly squeezed lemon juice
Salt
Freshly ground black pepper

1. Toast the bread. Spread 1 teaspoon of the canna-butter on each slice.

2. Place 2 slices of tomato on each piece of toast, if using.

3. Toss the avocado with the lemon juice and divide the slices between the 2 pieces of toast.

4. Season with salt and pepper.

5. Serve warm.

6. Store the remaining serving in an airtight container in the refrigerator for up to 2 days. Enjoy the second serving chilled or at room temperature.

- -

It is sometimes difficult to find ripe avocados. Place an under-ripe avocado in a brown paper bag to hasten ripening. The ethylene gas produced by the fruit will help it ripen, usually within 3 to 4 days.

PER SERVING Calories: 212; Total Fat: 19.7g; Saturated Fat: 4.2g; Cholesterol: 0mg; Carbohydrates: 10.0g; Fiber: 7.1g; Protein: 2.2g

SCRAMBLED EGGS
WITH CARAMELIZED ONIONS AND CHEESE

GLUTEN-FREE | NUT-FREE | SOY-FREE | SUGAR-FREE | VEGETARIAN

These scrambled eggs can be the centerpiece of your brunch table, but this egg dish is pretty fabulous on its own.

MAKES 2 SERVINGS

Prep time: 10 minutes
Cook time: 25 minutes

 DOSAGE TEST

Start with half of a serving and wait 4 hours to fully assess your reaction to its strength and effects.

1 tablespoon butter
2 teaspoons canna-butter (page 106)
½ cup thinly sliced onion
4 large eggs, beaten
½ cup shredded cheese (any type)
Salt
Freshly ground black pepper

1. In a medium nonstick skillet, heat the butters over medium heat. Add the onion, and sauté for 13 to 15 minutes, until the onions are browned and caramelized.

2. Add the eggs and cook for 6 to 8 minutes, stirring until set.

3. Add the cheese and continue to cook for 3 to 5 minutes, until the cheese is almost melted. Season with salt and pepper.

4. Serve warm.

5. Store the remaining serving in an airtight container in the refrigerator for up to 2 days. Reheat in the microwave on low power for 2 minutes or until warm.

- -

For some greens with this breakfast scramble, add a cup of fresh spinach to the onions before adding the eggs.

PER SERVING Calories: 206; Total Fat: 15.7g; Saturated Fat: 6.8g; Cholesterol: 367mg; Carbohydrates: 3.5g; Fiber: 0.6g; Protein: 13g

BAKED EGGS IN AVOCADO

GLUTEN-FREE | NUT-FREE | SOY-FREE | SUGAR-FREE | VEGETARIAN

With two healthy fats—egg yolk and avocado—this meal can be made in just minutes. Trust us, it is a great combo.

MAKES 2 SERVINGS

Prep time: 10 minutes
Cook time: 15 minutes

 DOSAGE TEST

Start with half of a serving and wait 4 hours to fully assess your reaction to its strength and effects.

1 large avocado
1 tablespoon freshly squeezed lemon juice
2 teaspoons canna-butter (page 106)
2 medium eggs, at room temperature
Salt
Freshly ground black pepper
1 scallion, chopped (optional)
¼ bunch cilantro, chopped (optional)
¼ cup shredded Cheddar cheese (optional)
2 tablespoons salsa (optional)

1. Preheat the oven to 340ºF.

2. Cut the avocado in half, remove the pit, and cover all exposed areas with the lemon juice. Place on a baking sheet, cut sides up.

3. Enlarge the cavities in the avocado to accommodate the eggs. Eat what you remove! Add a teaspoon of canna-butter to each avocado half.

4. Crack the eggs, placing one in the center of each avocado. Sprinkle with salt and pepper.

5. Place the baking sheet in the oven and bake until the eggs are set, 12 to 16 minutes, depending on how cooked you like your eggs.

6. Remove, place the avocados on a plate, and top with any of the optional garnishes.

7. Store the remaining serving in an airtight container in the refrigerator for up to 2 days. Enjoy cold as a leftover.

- -

If you want to indulge yourself, top the baked egg with some sour cream and bacon bits.

PER SERVING Calories: 303; Total Fat: 27.8g; Saturated Fat: 8g; Cholesterol: 174mg; Carbohydrates: 9.1g; Fiber: 6.8g; Protein: 7.5g

SALMON
WITH SHREDDED CARROTS

GLUTEN-FREE | NUT-FREE | SUGAR-FREE

If care is taken, salmon microwaves beautifully. The salmon stays moist in the waxed paper bags, which contain its juices and allow all the flavors to mingle.

MAKES 2 SERVINGS

Prep time: 10 minutes
Cook time: 6 minutes

Required Equipment
Waxed paper bags

 DOSAGE TEST

Start with half of a serving and wait 4 hours to fully assess your reaction to its strength and effects.

2 (5- to 6-ounce) salmon fillets
¼ cup snow peas
¼ cup peas
¼ cup shredded carrots
1 tablespoon orange juice
2 teaspoons canna-oil (page 105), at room temperature
1 teaspoon soy sauce
4 orange slices

1. Rinse and pat dry the salmon fillets and place each in a waxed paper bag, leaving the bag open.

2. In a small bowl, combine the snow peas, peas, carrots, orange juice, canna-oil, and soy sauce. Stir well.

3. Divide the mixture in half and pour over the salmon, inside each bag.

4. Place 2 orange slices on top of each salmon fillet.

5. Fold the bags closed under the fish.

6. Place the bags on a microwave-safe plate in a 1200-watt microwave and cook on high for 6 minutes.

7. Open the bags carefully and transfer the salmon and contents to a dish.

▶

SALMON
WITH SHREDDED CARROTS

8. Serve warm.

9. Store the remaining serving in an airtight container in the refrigerator for up to 2 days. Reheat in the microwave on low power for 2 minutes or until warm, or enjoy chilled.

When salmon is overcooked, this normally moist fish becomes unpleasantly dry. It's still safe to eat (and incredibly tasty) if it's still a little pink in the center.

PER SERVING Calories: 313; Total Fat: 15.4g; Saturated Fat: 1.9g; Cholesterol: 75mg; Carbohydrates: 8.9g; Fiber: 2.8g; Protein: 35g

STUFFED SWEET POTATO

GLUTEN-FREE | SOY-FREE | VEGAN

Sweet potatoes, rich and full of flavor, are among the healthiest foods you can eat. This stuffed sweet potato is a delightful addition to any meal.

MAKES 2 SERVINGS

Prep time: 10 minutes
Cook time: 15 minutes

 DOSAGE TEST

Start with half of a serving and wait 4 hours to fully assess your reaction to its strength and effects.

1 sweet potato, baked until tender
2 tablespoons orange juice
2 teaspoons canna-oil (page 105)
1 teaspoon agave
¼ cup golden raisins
2 tablespoons chopped walnuts

1. Preheat the oven to 340°F.

2. Cut the baked sweet potato in half and scoop out the filling.

3. Transfer the filling to a medium bowl and place the sweet potato halves cut-side up on a baking sheet.

4. Add the orange juice, canna-oil, agave, and raisins to the bowl and mix well.

5. Divide the filling between the sweet potato halves and spread evenly. Sprinkle the walnuts on top.

6. Bake for 15 to 17 minutes.

7. Serve warm.

8. Store the remaining serving in an airtight container in the refrigerator for up to 5 days. Reheat in the microwave on low power for 2 minutes or until warm, or enjoy chilled.

- -

If you haven't baked your sweet potato ahead of time, cook it in the microwave. Prick the skin of the potato with a fork and cover with a damp paper towel. Microwave on high for 5 minutes.

PER SERVING Calories: 209; Total Fat: 5g; Saturated Fat: 0g; Cholesterol: 0mg; Carbohydrates: 39.7g; Fiber: 4.6g; Protein: 4.6g

COUSCOUS
WITH CAULIFLOWER AND RAISINS

NUT-FREE | SOY-FREE | SUGAR-FREE

Couscous is easy to make and pairs well with many different foods and flavors. This particular combination is a favorite.

MAKES 2 SERVINGS

Prep time: 10 minutes
Cook time: 12 minutes

 DOSAGE TEST

Start with half of a serving and wait 4 hours to fully assess your reaction to its strength and effects.

1 tablespoon olive oil
2 teaspoons canna-oil (page 105)
1 small onion, peeled and chopped
1 small head cauliflower, cored and chopped
Pinch salt
⅔ cup extra-rich canned chicken broth
⅓ cup yellow raisins
⅓ cup whole-wheat couscous

1. In a medium saucepan, heat the oils over medium heat. Add the onion, cauliflower, and salt, and sauté for 5 to 7 minutes.

2. Add the broth, raisins, and couscous, and bring to a boil.

3. Immediately remove from the heat, cover, and let stand for 5 minutes.

4. Serve warm.

5. Store the remaining serving in an airtight container in the refrigerator for up to 3 days. Reheat in the microwave on low power for 2 minutes or until warm, or enjoy chilled.

- -

If you have leftovers, warm and serve them topped with a fried egg for a tasty breakfast treat.

PER SERVING Calories: 242; Total Fat: 13.2g; Saturated Fat: 1.8g; Cholesterol: 0mg; Carbohydrates: 27.6g; Fiber: 3.8g; Protein: 7g

THREE-MUSHROOM STEW
WITH PASTA

NUT-FREE | SOY-FREE | SUGAR-FREE | VEGAN

Mushrooms and rosemary are a winning combination. This recipe is particularly spectacular in the fall when there are beautiful fresh mushrooms at the farmers' markets.

MAKES 6 SERVINGS

Prep time: 10 minutes
Cook time: 20 minutes

 DOSAGE TEST

Start with half of a serving and wait 4 hours to fully assess your reaction to its strength and effects.

1 pound pasta (any type)
2 tablespoons canna-oil (page 105)
1 tablespoon olive oil
2 leeks, chopped
2 medium carrots, peeled and sliced
2 garlic cloves, thinly sliced
2 pounds assorted mushrooms, cut into uniform pieces
2 tablespoons chopped fresh rosemary
½ teaspoon salt
½ teaspoon freshly ground black pepper

1. Cook the pasta according to the package directions. Drain the pasta and transfer to a large bowl.

2. In a large skillet, heat the oils over medium heat. Add the leeks and carrots, and sauté for 8 to 10 minutes until tender.

3. Add the garlic, stir to combine, and transfer the mixture to a medium bowl.

4. Place the mushrooms in the hot skillet and cook for 8 to 10 minutes over medium heat, until the liquid has evaporated and the mushrooms begin to brown.

5. Add the rosemary, salt, and pepper, and return the vegetables to the skillet. Stir to combine.

▶

THREE-MUSHROOM STEW
WITH PASTA

6. Divide the cooked pasta into 6 portions, and top each with an equal portion of the mushroom-vegetable mixture.

7. Serve warm.

8. Store the remaining servings in an airtight container in the refrigerator for up to 4 days. Reheat in the microwave on low power for 2 minutes or until warm.

- -

Remember to let the mushrooms release their liquid. Browning them adds an earthiness that is an important part of this dish. When it comes to the leeks, do not use the tough green tops.

PER SERVING Calories: 311; Total Fat: 9.0g; Saturated Fat: 1g; Cholesterol: 55mg; Carbohydrates: 48.7g; Fiber: 1.6g; Protein: 9.3g

BAKED RICE CASSEROLE

GLUTEN-FREE | NUT-FREE | SOY-FREE | SUGAR-FREE | VEGETARIAN

A baked casserole is one of the ultimate comfort foods. You can vary the vegetables and the cheese in this recipe to suit your taste. If you want to include some protein, adding cooked chicken or lean ground beef to the casserole before baking is as easy as can be.

MAKES 4 SERVINGS

Prep time: 15 minutes
Cook time: 35 minutes

 DOSAGE TEST

Start with half of a serving and wait 4 hours to fully assess your reaction to its strength and effects.

Vegetable cooking spray
4 teaspoons canna-butter (page 106)
1 small onion, chopped
1 bell pepper, seeded and chopped
1 (10-ounce) package frozen chopped spinach, thawed and squeezed of liquid
1 cup low-fat milk
2 eggs
2 cups shredded Cheddar cheese, divided
3 cups cooked brown or white rice
Pinch salt
Freshly ground black pepper

1. Preheat the oven to 340°F. Coat a large casserole dish with cooking spray and set aside.

2. In a large sauté pan or skillet, heat the canna-butter over medium-low heat. Add the onion and bell pepper and cook until softened, 5 to 7 minutes. Add the spinach and cook for 3 to 4 minutes. Remove from the heat and set aside.

3. In a large bowl, combine the milk and eggs and mix well. Add 1½ cups of cheese, the rice, and the cooked vegetables and mix well. Season with salt and pepper and mix again.

4. Transfer the mixture to the prepared casserole dish. Top with the remaining ½ cup of cheese and bake for about 25 minutes, or until the cheese is melted and golden brown.

5. Store any remaining servings in an airtight container in the refrigerator for up to 4 days. Reheat in the microwave on low power for 2 minutes or until warm.

- -

Many other delicious and healthy ancient grains would work well in this recipe, such as farro, brown rice, quinoa, or teff.

PER SERVING Calories: 362; Total Fat: 11.9g; Saturated Fat: 6.4g; Cholesterol: 109mg; Carbohydrates: 39.8g; Fiber: 3.0g; Protein: 23.9g

SO-GOOD FRITTATA

GLUTEN-FREE | NUT-FREE | SOY-FREE | SUGAR-FREE | VEGETARIAN

A wonderful one-dish meal, frittatas are great for breakfast, lunch, or dinner. The protein-rich eggs and cheese, along with plenty of vegetables, will fill and nourish you.

MAKES 4 SERVINGS

Prep time: 10 minutes
Cook time: 25 minutes

 DOSAGE TEST

Start with half of a serving and wait 4 hours to fully assess your reaction to its strength and effects.

Vegetable cooking spray
1 tablespoon plus 1 teaspoon canna-oil (page 105)
1 cup chopped bell pepper
1 cup corn kernels, fresh or frozen
½ cup chopped scallions
6 large eggs
½ teaspoon salt
½ teaspoon freshly ground black pepper
3 cups fresh spinach, rinsed and dried
2 ounces goat cheese, crumbled
Pinch smoked paprika

1. Preheat the oven to 340ºF.

2. Lightly coat a large ovenproof pan with the cooking spray, then add the canna-oil. Heat over medium heat.

3. Add the bell pepper, and sauté for 6 to 7 minutes until tender.

4. Add the corn and scallions, and sauté for 4 to 5 minutes until tender. Remove from heat.

5. In a medium bowl, beat the eggs. Add the salt and pepper and stir well.

6. Return the pan with the vegetables back to the heat. Add the spinach and cook for 4 to 5 minutes until wilted.

7. Pour the eggs into the pan, and evenly distribute the vegetables.

8. Spread the goat cheese over the mixture, and place the pan in the oven.

9. Bake for 8 to 10 minutes until set and golden brown.

10. Sprinkle with the paprika, and cut into 4 wedges.

11. Serve warm.

12. Store the remaining servings in an airtight container in the refrigerator for up to 5 days. Reheat in the microwave on low power for 2 minutes or until warm.

- -

This dish is also terrific at room temperature and even chilled.

PER SERVING Calories: 183; Total Fat: 12.6g; Saturated Fat: 5.8g; Cholesterol: 294mg; Carbohydrates: 3.4g; Fiber: 0.9g; Protein: 14.2g

PAN-ROASTED CAULIFLOWER
WITH CARROTS, SWEET POTATO, AND ZUCCHINI

GLUTEN-FREE | NUT-FREE | SOY-FREE | VEGETARIAN

This is a simple, earthy, and nutritious roasted vegetable plate. It can accompany a piece of fish or chicken, but it is delicious on its own.

MAKES 4 SERVINGS

Prep time: 15 minutes
Cook time: 40 minutes

 DOSAGE TEST

Start with half of a serving and wait 4 hours to fully assess your reaction to its strength and effects.

1 medium head cauliflower, cored and broken into florets
4 thin carrots, peeled
1 sweet potato, peeled and cubed
2 zucchini, cut into thick slices
1 red onion, peeled and cut in wedges
2 tablespoons olive oil
4 teaspoons canna-oil (page 105)
1 tablespoon maple syrup
1 teaspoon garlic salt
½ teaspoon freshly ground black pepper
1 cup plain yogurt or sour cream

1. Preheat the oven to 325ºF.

2. In a cast iron pan or baking dish, toss together the cauliflower, carrots, sweet potato, zucchini, and onion.

3. In a small bowl, combine the oils and maple syrup.

4. Pour the oil-syrup mixture over the vegetables, add the garlic salt and pepper, and toss until the vegetables are well coated.

5. Bake for 35 to 40 minutes until the vegetables are fork-tender.

6. Serve warm. When ready to eat, top each serving with ¼ cup of the yogurt or sour cream.

7. Store the remaining servings in an airtight container in the refrigerator for up to 3 days. Reheat in the microwave on low power for 2 minutes or until warm. (Add the yogurt or sour cream only when ready to eat.)

Feel free to experiment with different vegetables to suit your taste; you can't go wrong. You can use leftovers in an omelet, maybe with some shredded Cheddar cheese.

PER SERVING Calories: 162; Total Fat: 11.9g; Saturated Fat: 1.4g; Cholesterol: 0mg; Carbohydrates: 14.1g; Fiber: 2.2g; Protein: 1.6g

SPINACH, AVOCADO, AND LIME SMOOTHIE

GLUTEN-FREE | VEGAN

This refreshing smoothie is a meal in itself. Nutritious and delicious, it's easy to prepare.

MAKES 2 SERVINGS

Prep time: 10 minutes

Required Equipment
Blender

 DOSAGE TEST

Start with half of a serving and wait 4 hours to fully assess your reaction to its strength and effects.

2 cups almond milk
1 cup packed fresh spinach
½ avocado, peeled, pitted, and sliced
½ cup soft tofu
2 tablespoons freshly squeezed lime juice
2 tablespoons coconut sugar
2 teaspoons canna-oil (page 105)

1. In a blender, combine all the ingredients and purée for 1 to 2 minutes until smooth.

2. Serve immediately.

3. Store the remaining serving in an airtight container in the refrigerator for up to 3 days. Blend again before serving.

- -

For a richer meal, you can substitute coconut milk for the almond milk. To make this an extra-special treat, run a lime wedge around the rim of the glass and dip the glass in coconut sugar before pouring.

PER SERVING Calories: 300; Total Fat: 24.2g; Saturated Fat: 8g; Cholesterol: 0mg; Carbohydrates: 9.2g; Fiber: 7.1g; Protein: 2.3g

SKILLET STIR-FRY CHICKEN
WITH VEGETABLES

GLUTEN-FREE | NUT-FREE | SUGAR-FREE

You don't need a wok to make a great stir-fry. A skillet can work just as well. There are lots of delicious vegetables in this dish, along with a good dose of protein.

MAKES 2 SERVINGS

Prep time: 10 minutes
Cook time: 20 minutes

 DOSAGE TEST

Start with half of a serving and wait 4 hours to fully assess your reaction to its strength and effects.

8 cups water
2 cups broccoli florets
1 large carrot, sliced
1 cup trimmed, halved green beans
1 tablespoon canola oil
1 large boneless, skinless chicken breast, cut into chunks
3 tablespoons hoisin sauce
2 teaspoons canna-oil (page 105)
½ teaspoon ground ginger
Salt
Freshly ground black pepper

1. In a medium saucepan, bring the water to a boil. Add the broccoli, carrot, and green beans, and cook for 6 minutes over medium heat. Drain and run the vegetables under cold water.

2. In a large skillet, heat the canola oil. Add the chicken, and sauté over medium heat for 7 to 9 minutes until cooked through.

3. Add the vegetables to the skillet and cook for an additional 4 to 5 minutes over medium heat.

4. In a small bowl, combine the hoisin sauce, canna-oil, and ginger.

5. Add the sauce to the pan, and stir to coat.

6. Season with salt and pepper.

▶

7. Serve warm.

8. Store the remaining serving in an airtight container in the refrigerator for up to 2 days. Reheat in the microwave on low power for 2 minutes or until warm.

- -

You can serve this stir-fry over brown or white rice if you'd like. This recipe also works well with shrimp, beef slices, or tofu cubes in place of the chicken.

PER SERVING Calories: 149; Total Fat: 11.9g; Saturated Fat: 1.1g; Cholesterol: 0mg; Carbohydrates: 9.9g; Fiber: 3.3g; Protein: 2.9g

GRILLED CHICKEN AND CORN

GLUTEN-FREE | NUT-FREE | SOY-FREE | SUGAR-FREE

Sometimes throwing something on the grill is the easiest way to go. This dish cooks up in no time, and is a great way to showcase fresh corn.

MAKES 4 SERVINGS

Prep time: 30 minutes, plus 1 hour marinating time
Cook time: 10 minutes

Required equipment
8 (4-inch) wood skewers

 DOSAGE TEST

Start with half of a serving and wait 4 hours to fully assess your reaction to its strength and effects.

¼ cup olive oil
4 teaspoons canna-oil (page 105)
¼ cup chopped fresh cilantro
1 garlic clove, minced
3 boneless, skinless chicken breasts, cut into chunks
4 ears of corn, cut into 1-inch pieces
½ pint whole cherry tomatoes
4 scallions, cut into 1-inch pieces
Salt
Freshly ground black pepper

1. Preheat the grill to medium heat. Soak 8 wood skewers in water for 30 minutes.

2. In a small bowl, combine the oils, cilantro, and garlic for the marinade.

3. Place the chicken in a separate bowl, and cover the chicken with half of the marinade. Marinate for 1 hour.

4. Thread the presoaked skewers with the chicken, corn, tomatoes, and scallions. Salt and pepper the skewers.

5. Brush the skewers with half of the remaining marinade and place on the grill.

6. Cook on medium heat until the chicken turns golden brown and the vegetables are cooked, 7 to 10 minutes. Turn halfway through the cooking time.

➤

GRILLED CHICKEN AND CORN

CONTINUED

7. Brush the skewers with the remaining marinade before serving.

8. Store any remaining servings in an airtight container in the refrigerator for up to 2 days. Reheat in the microwave on low power for 2 minutes or until warm.

- -

You can replace the chicken with cubed extra-firm tofu or shrimp.

PER SERVING Calories: 432; Total Fat: 25.6g; Saturated Fat: 4.7g; Cholesterol: 93mg; Carbohydrates: 20g; Fiber: 3.2g; Protein: 33.2g

EASY MACARONI AND CHEESE

NUT-FREE | SOY-FREE | SUGAR-FREE | VEGETARIAN

Macaroni and cheese is a good go-to when you're feeling a little under the weather. This recipe calls for Cheddar, but it's also tasty with other cheeses. You can add some chopped cooked broccoli or other vegetable to the dish once the cheese has melted. For a lighter version, use skim milk and reduce the amount of butter and cheese.

MAKES 2 SERVINGS

Prep time: 10 minutes
Cook time: 15 minutes

 DOSAGE TEST

Start with half of a serving and wait 4 hours to fully assess your reaction to its strength and effects.

8 ounces macaroni
¼ cup (½ stick) butter
2 teaspoons canna-butter (page 106)
3 tablespoons all-purpose flour
¼ teaspoon salt
¼ teaspoon freshly ground black pepper
2 cups whole milk
2 cups shredded Cheddar cheese

1. Cook the macaroni according to the package directions. Drain the macaroni and transfer to a medium bowl.

2. In a medium saucepan, melt the butters over medium heat.

3. Stir in the flour, salt, and pepper.

4. Slowly add the milk, stirring constantly for 7 to 9 minutes until bubbly.

5. Add the cheese, and stir until completely melted.

6. Add the cheese mixture to the pasta, and stir until completely coated.

7. Serve warm.

8. Store the remaining serving in an airtight container in the refrigerator for up to 3 days. Reheat in the microwave on low power for 2 minutes or until warm.

- -

Make some extra pasta, toss it with a little oil, and keep it in the refrigerator to use in your recipes. If you need a quick meal, just heat up a serving, add 2 teaspoons of canna-butter and some grated Parmesan cheese, and voilà!

PER SERVING Calories: 445; Total Fat: 33.4g; Saturated Fat: 21.1g; Cholesterol: 97mg; Carbohydrates: 23.5g; Fiber: 0g; Protein: 37.2g

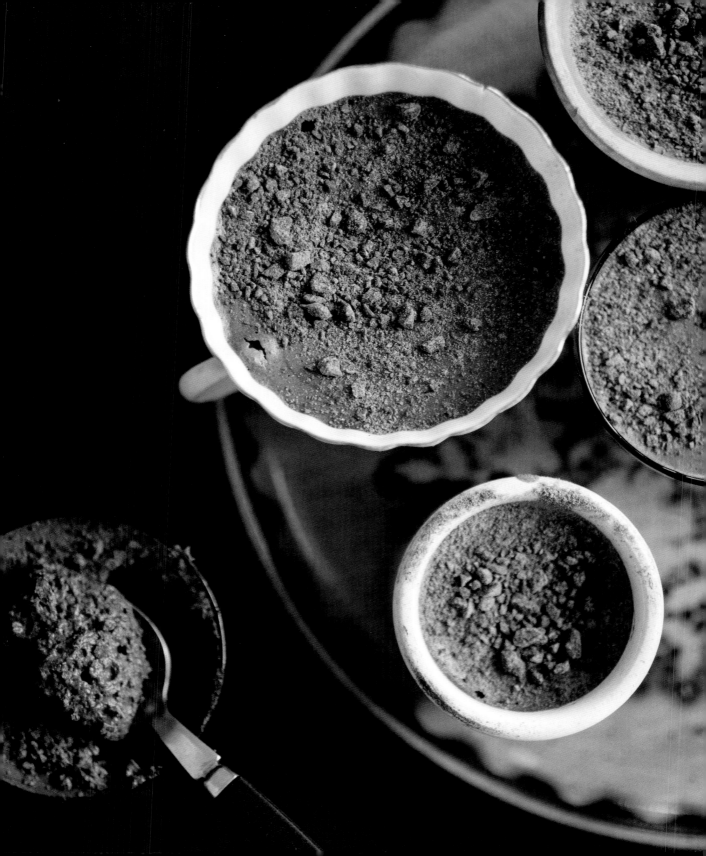

SWEET CANNABIS EDIBLES

SWEET TREATS DON'T have to be unhealthy. Using fruits and natural sweeteners like honey and maple syrup, you can enjoy desserts that are loaded with wonderful nutrients and other health benefits. Starting with canna-butter (page 106) or canna-oil (page 105), whipping these treats up will be a piece of cake. All of these recipes are easy to prepare at home. By making them in your own kitchen, you will be sure of the dosage and can alter the dish to suit your health needs.

Required Equipment

Most recipes require no special equipment other than a stove top, an oven, a baking sheet, and a sauté pan or saucepan. Besides these basic kitchen tools, we recommend the following items for some of the recipes.

Blender—This kitchen appliance is used to blend, purée, and liquefy. You can use a standard blender or an immersion blender. You can find a blender online or at your local kitchen and home supply store.

Double Boiler—This is essentially two pots that fit together, one on top of the other. The bottom pot is filled with water and the top pot is filled with ingredients that shouldn't receive direct heat. If you don't have a double boiler, you can place a heat-safe mixing bowl over a saucepan of water. The upper bowl should not touch the water in the saucepan.

Electric Mixer—This kitchen tool makes the work of stirring, beating, and whisking much easier. You can use either a hand mixer or a stand mixer. You can find a mixer online or at your kitchen and home supply store.

Food Processor—This versatile machine is used for slicing, shredding, grinding, puréeing, and blending. You can find one online or at your local kitchen and home supply store.

Ice Pop Mold—Great for making frozen treats at home, ice pop molds consist of a base, molds, and sticks or handles. Ice pop molds can be found online or at your kitchen and home supply store.

Slow Cooker—This large electric pot is a convenient way to cook foods over a long period of time. You can find one online or at your kitchen and home supply store.

THOUGHTS AND EXPERIENCES

I am a school teacher with multiple sclerosis, and I've worked with doctors to find a treatment to relieve my pain. I've tried so many pills, but none really worked. When my doctor suggested marijuana, I laughed, thinking he was joking. But he shared studies and wrote a recommendation for an Oregon Medical Marijuana Program (OMMP) card.

I got my card, and over the past year, I have been working with a dispensary to find the right type of marijuana for me. It definitely helps, especially with my terrible headaches and spasms. Recently, I tried a CBD strain that doesn't get me high at all and provides relief throughout the day. It also helps lift my mood when I feel down, which tends to happen all too often with my condition.

Over summer vacation, when I'm not teaching, I feel better because there is less stress and restrictions on my medication. I eat one or two edibles every day, and I feel like a different person. Because it has been a huge relief for me, it makes sense that people with health issues should be able to try it. I wish I could talk about medical marijuana more openly. I do think attitudes are shifting. Hopefully, it will soon be legal everywhere. Then we can just relax.
—**Mia M.**, Oregon

DARK CHOCOLATE GRANOLA CLUSTERS

NUT-FREE | SOY-FREE | VEGETARIAN

Chocolate, cannabis, and granola (three nutritional superheroes) are just meant to be together. Dark chocolate has many health benefits, and granola is packed with fiber and essential nutrients. Use your favorite store-bought or homemade granola in this recipe.

MAKES 36 CLUSTERS

[4 clusters = 1 serving]
Prep time: 5 minutes, plus
    1 hour cooling time
Cook time: 10 minutes

Required Equipment
Double boiler

 DOSAGE TEST

Start with half of a serving and wait 4 hours to fully assess your reaction to its strength and effects.

1¼ cups dark chocolate melting wafers
3 tablespoons canna-oil (page 105)
⅔ cup granola
1 tablespoon flaxseed

1. Prepare your work surface by spreading out a piece of parchment paper or aluminum foil.

2. In a double boiler, combine the chocolate and canna-oil. Heat over medium heat, stirring as needed, until fully melted.

3. Remove from the heat, and stir in the granola and flaxseed until well combined.

4. Drop the chocolate-granola mixture by tablespoons onto the parchment paper, spacing the clusters evenly apart.

5. Allow to cool for at least 1 hour.

6. Store the clusters in an airtight container at room temperature for up to 1 week or in the refrigerator for up to 2 weeks.

- -

If the chocolate gets too hot or water gets into the bowl, the chocolate can seize up and get lumpy, so be careful. You can substitute dried fruit or nuts for the granola. Or, if you want to feel like a kid again, add a handful of crumbled graham crackers and mini marshmallows for a s'more delight!

PER SERVING Calories: 230; Total Fat: 18.2g; Saturated Fat: 10.7g; Cholesterol: 0mg; Carbohydrates: 28.3g; Fiber: 1.8g; Protein: 4.9g

OVERNIGHT BAKED FRENCH TOAST

NUT-FREE | SOY-FREE | VEGETARIAN

Wake up and pop this toast in the oven for a great way to start the day. Serve with maple syrup or a dollop of vanilla yogurt.

MAKES 6 SLICES

[3 slices = 1 serving]
Prep time: 10 minutes
Cook time: 50 minutes, plus overnight refrigeration

 DOSAGE TEST

Start with half of a serving and wait 4 hours to fully assess your reaction to its strength and effects.

1 teaspoon butter
3 eggs
½ cup milk
1 tablespoon sugar
2 teaspoons canna-butter (page 106), melted
1 teaspoon vanilla extract
Pinch salt
Pinch ground cinnamon
6 slices day-old bread, torn

1. Butter a baking dish and set aside.

2. In a medium bowl, combine the eggs, milk, sugar, canna-butter, vanilla, salt, and cinnamon.

3. Add the bread, combine, and turn into the buttered dish.

4. Cover with plastic wrap and chill overnight in the refrigerator.

5. Preheat the oven to 340ºF.

6. Bake for 45 to 50 minutes until set and golden brown.

7. Serve warm.

8. Store the remaining serving in an airtight container in the refrigerator for up to 2 days. Reheat in the microwave on low power for 2 minutes or until warm.

You can also make French toast muffins by dividing the mixture into 5 or 6 muffin tins and baking for the same length of time.

PER SERVING Calories: 171; Total Fat: 9.7g; Saturated Fat: 4.0g; Cholesterol: 256mg; Carbohydrates: 9.9g; Fiber: 0g; Protein: 10.3g

COCONUT BREAKFAST PUDDING

GLUTEN-FREE | NUT-FREE | SOY-FREE | SUGAR-FREE | VEGAN

This filling breakfast is a coconut lover's dream come true. It's also healthy and satisfying. If you are a coconut fan, this breakfast pudding will be a real treat for you!

MAKES 2 SERVINGS

Prep time: 5 minutes
Cook time: 15 minutes, plus
   overnight refrigeration

 DOSAGE TEST

Start with half of a serving and wait 4 hours to fully assess your reaction to its strength and effects.

¾ cup old-fashioned gluten-free oats
½ cup unsweetened shredded coconut
2 cups water
1¼ cups coconut milk
2 teaspoons canna-oil (page 105)
½ teaspoon ground cinnamon
1 banana, sliced

1. In a medium bowl, combine the oats, coconut, and water. Cover and chill overnight.

2. Transfer the mixture to a small saucepan. Add the milk, canna-oil, and cinnamon, and simmer for about 12 minutes over medium heat.

3. Remove from the heat, and let stand for 5 minutes.

4. Divide between 2 bowls and top with the banana slices.

5. Store the remaining serving in an airtight container in the refrigerator for up to 4 days. Enjoy the second serving chilled or at room temperature.

- -

If you are in the mood for an even tastier treat, sauté the banana slices in a little butter and brown sugar before topping the pudding.

PER SERVING Calories: 127; Total Fat: 34.4g; Saturated Fat: 6.2g; Cholesterol: 0mg; Carbohydrates: 34.7g; Fiber: 9.8g; Protein: 13.2g

CHIA SEED PUDDING

GLUTEN-FREE | SOY-FREE | SUGAR-FREE | VEGAN

This healthy, delicious vegan pudding is a great source of omega-3 fatty acids, calcium, and antioxidants. When combined with liquid, chia seeds thicken to a gel-like consistency. With a little planning, it takes just a few minutes to pull together for a satisfying breakfast or dessert.

MAKES 4 SERVINGS

Prep time: 10 minutes, plus
  overnight refrigeration

Required Equipment
Blender

 DOSAGE TEST

Start with half of a serving and wait 4 hours to fully assess your reaction to its strength and effects.

1½ cups almond milk
8 dates, pitted and chopped
⅓ cup chia seeds
¼ cup unsweetened cocoa powder
4 teaspoons canna-oil (page 105)
½ teaspoon ground cinnamon

1. In a medium bowl, combine all the ingredients. Stir well.

2. Cover with plastic wrap and chill in the refrigerator overnight.

3. Transfer the mixture to a blender and pulse several times until coarse and uniform.

4. Pour the mixture into individual pudding bowls.

5. Cover the remaining servings with plastic wrap and store in the refrigerator for up to a week.

- -

You can substitute coconut milk, soy milk, or dairy milk for the almond milk. When the chia seeds are soaked in liquid, they become gelatinous little balls, similar to tapioca pudding. When the chia seeds are processed in a blender, they lose their structure and their gelatinous properties are more evenly distributed throughout the pudding. If you would like to keep the tapioca-like texture of soaked chia seeds, simply omit the blender step.

PER SERVING Calories: 114; Total Fat: 6.6g; Saturated Fat: 4.5g; Cholesterol: 0mg; Carbohydrates: 16.3g; Fiber: 3.6g; Protein: 1.9g

SIMPLE RICE PUDDING
WITH RAISINS AND APRICOTS

GLUTEN-FREE | NUT-FREE | SOY-FREE | VEGETARIAN

Rice pudding could easily fall into the Top 10 Comfort Foods category. Warm or cold, this pudding is a creamy, comforting treat.

MAKES 6 SERVINGS

Prep time: 5 minutes
Cook time: 25 minutes

 DOSAGE TEST

Start with half of a serving and wait 4 hours to fully assess your reaction to its strength and effects.

3 cups whole milk
3 cups cooked white rice
2 tablespoons canna-butter (page 106)
½ cup raisins
½ cup chopped dried apricots
⅓ cup brown sugar
¼ teaspoon ground cinnamon
2 teaspoons vanilla extract

1. In a medium saucepan, combine the milk, rice, canna-butter, raisins, apricots, sugar, and cinnamon. Bring to a boil, then immediately reduce the heat.

2. Simmer gently over low heat for 25 minutes or until the rice is tender.

3. Stir in the vanilla.

4. Serve warm.

5. Store the remaining servings in an airtight container in the refrigerator for up to a week. Reheat in the microwave on low heat for 2 minutes or until warm, or enjoy chilled.

- -

To prevent burning, cook the pudding over low heat. If you want plain rice pudding, you can leave out the dried fruit.

PER SERVING Calories: 319; Total Fat: 7.9g; Saturated Fat: 4.7g; Cholesterol: 25mg; Carbohydrates: 55.9g; Fiber: 1.4g; Protein: 8.5g

ORANGE AND GINGER ICE POPS

GLUTEN-FREE | NUT-FREE | SOY-FREE | VEGETARIAN

Refreshing and nutritious, homemade cannabis ice pops are a great treat to have in the freezer. Sucking on an ice pop is an excellent way to medicate and soothe a dry mouth.

MAKES 6 ICE POPS

[1 ice pop = 1 serving]
Prep time: 10 minutes, plus
  2 hours freezing time

Required Equipment

Blender
Ice pop molds

 DOSAGE TEST

Start with half of a serving and wait 4 hours to fully assess your reaction to its strength and effects.

2 cups orange juice
2 tablespoons canna-oil (page 105)
2 tablespoons honey
½ teaspoon ground ginger
¼ teaspoon ground turmeric

1. In a blender, combine all the ingredients, and pulse a few times.

2. Pour the mixture into 6 ice pop molds.

3. Freeze for at least 2 hours.

4. Store in the freezer in the molds for up to 1 month.

If you would like fruit in your pops, add a few pieces when you fill the molds. Raspberries or blueberries are the perfect size, but you can chop up any type of fruit you like into small pieces. After 20 minutes in the freezer, stir each ice pop once or twice to prevent the fruit from settling at the bottom.

PER SERVING Calories: 88; Total Fat: 4.7g; Saturated Fat: 3.9g; Cholesterol: 0mg; Carbohydrates: 11.7g; Fiber: 0g; Protein: 0g

CRANBERRY AND LIME ICE POPS

GLUTEN-FREE | NUT-FREE | SOY-FREE | VEGAN

A cannabis-infused favorite, these pops are light and a little tart. They are wonderful in the warm weather and for soothing dry mouth. For additional texture, you can add a small handful of dried cranberries to the ice pop molds before filling. Just remember to stir each ice pop once or twice after they've been in the freezer for 20 minutes to prevent the cranberries from settling at the bottom.

MAKES 6 SERVINGS

Prep time: 5 minutes, plus
   2 hours freezing time

Required Equipment
Blender
Ice pop molds

 DOSAGE TEST

Start with half of a serving and wait 4 hours to fully assess your reaction to its strength and effects.

1½ cups unsweetened cranberry juice
½ cup frozen limeade concentrate
3 tablespoons honey
2 tablespoons canna-oil (page 105)
1 tablespoon chia seeds

1. In a blender, combine all the ingredients, and pulse a few times.

2. Pour the mixture into 6 ice pop molds.

3. Freeze for at least 2 hours.

4. Store in the freezer in the molds for up to 1 month.

- -

If you don't like the tartness of cranberries or prefer a simple lime ice pop, just replace the unsweetened cranberry juice with an equal amount of water.

PER SERVING Calories: 91; Total Fat: 4.5g; Saturated Fat: 3.9g; Cholesterol: 0mg; Carbohydrates: 13.4g; Fiber: 0g; Protein: 0.1g

HEALING HERB-SPICED NUTS

GLUTEN-FREE | SOY-FREE | VEGETARIAN

Both turmeric and ginger have wonderful healing properties, including settling nausea, reducing inflammation, and lowering high blood pressure. And you thought nuts couldn't get any healthier!

MAKES 12 SERVINGS

Prep time: 10 minutes
Cook time: 25 minutes

 DOSAGE TEST

Start with half of a serving and wait 4 hours to fully assess your reaction to its strength and effects.

1 cup raw almonds
1 cup raw cashews
1 cup shelled peanuts
¼ cup canna-oil (page 105)
2 tablespoons honey
1 teaspoon ground turmeric
½ teaspoon ground ginger
½ teaspoon fenugreek seeds

1. Preheat the oven to 300ºF.

2. In a large bowl, combine all the ingredients. Toss until the nuts are evenly coated.

3. Spread out the nuts on a baking sheet.

4. Roast for 20 to 25 minutes, turning occasionally.

5. Allow to cool before eating.

6. Store in an airtight container at room temperature for up to 2 weeks or in the freezer for up to 2 months.

- -

Although the nuts may seem a bit oily when they first come out of the oven, this won't be an issue when they are fully cooled.

PER SERVING Calories: 231; Total Fat: 19.8g; Saturated Fat: 6.1g; Cholesterol: 0mg; Carbohydrates: 10.5g; Fiber: 2.5g; Protein: 6.6g

HONEY-BAKED ALMOND PEARS

GLUTEN-FREE | SOY-FREE | VEGETARIAN

Baked pears are a fall staple around our place. Sweetened with nutrient-rich maple syrup and topped with almonds, medicine never tasted so good!

MAKES 2 SERVINGS

Prep time: 10 minutes
Cook time: 30 minutes

 DOSAGE TEST

Start with half of a serving and wait 4 hours to fully assess your reaction to its strength and effects.

1 pear, halved and cored
4 teaspoons maple syrup
2 teaspoons canna-butter (page 106)
4 tablespoons sliced almonds

1. Heat the oven to 340°F.

2. Place the pear halves in a baking dish, cut-side up.

3. In the center of each pear, drizzle 2 teaspoons of maple syrup and add 1 teaspoon of canna-butter.

4. Bake for 15 minutes.

5. Carefully spread 2 tablespoons of almond slices over each half.

6. Continue baking for 15 minutes until golden brown and tender.

7. Serve warm.

8. Store the remaining serving in an airtight container in the refrigerator for up to 4 days. Reheat in the microwave on low heat for 2 minutes or until warm, or enjoy chilled.

- -

You can substitute walnuts, which also go well with pears, for the almonds. With a dollop of yogurt on top, this baked treat also makes for a homey breakfast.

PER SERVING Calories: 177; Total Fat: 9.9g; Saturated Fat: 2.9g; Cholesterol: 10mg; Carbohydrates: 22.1g; Fiber: 3.6g; Protein: 2.8g

APPLE CRISP

GLUTEN-FREE | NUT-FREE | SOY-FREE | VEGETARIAN

The aroma from this apple crisp baking in the oven is reason enough to make this glorious dish. Apples are packed with fiber and antioxidants and have been reported to help prevent diabetes and boost the immune system. Oats are said to help lower blood pressure as well as reduce the risk of certain types of cancer.

MAKES 2 SERVINGS

Prep time: 20 minutes
Cook time: 35 minutes

 DOSAGE TEST

Start with half of a serving and wait 4 hours to fully assess your reaction to its strength and effects.

2 apples, peeled, cored, and sliced
1 tablespoon orange juice
2 tablespoons brown sugar
2 tablespoons old-fashioned or quick gluten-free oats
2 tablespoons butter, melted
2 teaspoons canna-butter (page 106)
1 teaspoon vanilla extract
Pinch ground cinnamon

1. Preheat the oven to 325°F.

2. In a small baking dish, toss together the apple slices and orange juice.

3. In a medium bowl, combine the remaining ingredients. Stir well.

4. Sprinkle the sugar-oat mixture over the apples.

5. Bake for 30 to 35 minutes until the crust is golden brown and the apples are tender.

6. Serve warm.

7. Store the remaining serving in an airtight container in the refrigerator for up to 4 days. Reheat in the microwave on low heat for 2 minutes or until warm, or enjoy chilled.

- -

You can accompany this dish with a scoop of frozen yogurt or ice cream, if that's your style.

PER SERVING Calories: 230; Total Fat: 12.2g; Saturated Fat: 7.3g; Cholesterol: 31mg; Carbohydrates: 36.6g; Fiber: 5g; Protein: 1.4g

YOGURT WHIP
WITH PUREED SEASONAL FRUIT

GLUTEN-FREE | NUT-FREE | SOY-FREE | VEGETARIAN

Greek yogurt is thick and creamy and makes a totally yummy dessert. It is packed with protein, probiotics, potassium, and calcium. This is a treat you can happily enjoy on a daily basis.

MAKES 2 SERVINGS
Prep time: 15 minutes

Required Equipment
Electric mixer

 DOSAGE TEST

Start with half of a serving and wait 4 hours to fully assess your reaction to its strength and effects.

1½ cups plain Greek yogurt
2 tablespoons honey
2 teaspoons canna-oil (page 105)
½ teaspoon vanilla extract
1 cup puréed fresh berries (any type)

1. In a medium mixing bowl, combine the yogurt, honey, canna-oil, and vanilla.

2. Using an electric mixer or whisking by hand, beat the mixture until light and fluffy.

3. Fold the puréed berries into the yogurt.

4. Serve.

5. Store the remaining serving in an airtight container in the refrigerator for up to 4 days.

- -

If you want to use regular plain yogurt, first remove the excess liquid. Line a strainer with cheesecloth, place the strainer over a bowl, and empty the contents of the yogurt container into the lined strainer. Place it in the refrigerator overnight and discard the liquid in the morning.

PER SERVING Calories: 109; Total Fat: 1.2g; Saturated Fat: 1.0g; Cholesterol: 6mg; Carbohydrates: 15.8g; Fiber: 0g; Protein: 6.7g

DARK CHOCOLATE BLENDER PUDDING

GLUTEN-FREE | NUT-FREE | SOY-FREE | VEGETARIAN

With a velvety texture and a deep, rich taste, this pudding is almost too easy to be true! Keep in mind that this no-cook recipe calls for eggs. Although the hot coffee will slightly cook the eggs, you may not want to consume undercooked eggs if you have a weakened immune system.

MAKES 4 SERVINGS

Prep time: 10 minutes, plus 3 hours chill time

Required Equipment
Blender

 DOSAGE TEST

Start with half of a serving and wait 4 hours to fully assess your reaction to its strength and effects.

12 ounces dark chocolate chips
4 eggs, at room temperature*
4 teaspoons canna-butter (page 106), melted
2 teaspoons vanilla extract
1 teaspoon almond extract (optional)
Pinch salt
1 cup very hot coffee
2 ounces chopped dark chocolate (optional)

1. In a blender, combine the chocolate chips, eggs, canna-butter, vanilla, almond extract (if using), and salt. Pulse a few times to break the chocolate chips into pieces.

2. Remove the lid of the blender, and pour in the hot coffee, continuing to blend at a low speed. Replace the lid and blend for 2 minutes, until the pudding is silky smooth.

3. Pour the mixture into individual pudding bowls.

4. Allow to set for at least 3 hours in the refrigerator.

5. Before serving, top with chopped dark chocolate, if using.

6. Cover the remaining servings with plastic wrap and store in the refrigerator for up to 5 days.

- -

*Consuming raw or undercooked eggs may increase your risk of foodborne illness, especially if you have a weakened immune system.

PER SERVING Calories: 521; Total Fat: 33.4g; Saturated Fat: 21.4g; Cholesterol: 193mg; Carbohydrates: 51.3g; Fiber: 2.9g; Protein: 12.2g

STRAWBERRIES
WITH HONEY CREAM

GLUTEN-FREE | NUT-FREE | SOY-FREE | VEGETARIAN

When strawberries are in season, you might want to have this delicious dessert every night. Strawberries are an excellent source of fiber and essential nutrients, and Greek yogurt is packed with protein, probiotics, potassium, and calcium. Sweetened lightly with nutrient-rich honey, this flavorful combination is a soothing way to get the nutrients and medicine you need.

MAKES 2 SERVINGS

Prep time: 10 minutes

Required Equipment

Electric mixer

 DOSAGE TEST

Start with half of a serving and wait 4 hours to fully assess your reaction to its strength and effects.

1 cup plain, low-fat Greek yogurt
1 tablespoon honey
2 teaspoons canna-oil (page 105)
½ teaspoon vanilla extract
1 cup fresh strawberries, cleaned and sliced

1. In a small bowl, combine the yogurt, honey, canna-oil, and vanilla. Using an electric mixer or whisk, beat for 3 to 4 minutes until fluffy.

2. Divide the strawberries between 2 bowls, and top with equal portions of the honey cream.

3. Serve when ready to eat.

4. Store the remaining serving in an airtight container in the refrigerator for up to 3 days.

- -

You can use any type of fruit in place of the strawberries. The honey cream is also quite delicious with orange segments and walnuts.

PER SERVING Calories: 126; Total Fat: 5.8g; Saturated Fat: 4.8g; Cholesterol: 5mg; Carbohydrates: 11.7g; Fiber: 1.4 g; Protein: 5.3g

STEWED PRUNES

GLUTEN-FREE | NUT-FREE | SOY-FREE | VEGAN

The word "prunes" usually doesn't inspire joy or stimulate the appetite. If more people thought of them as dried plums, perhaps they could rise above their bad rap. Prunes are packed with fiber and sorbitol, which act as natural laxatives. They are also known for improving bone health, lowering cholesterol, and preventing diabetes.

MAKES 4 SERVINGS

Prep time: 5 minutes
Cook time: 30 minutes

 DOSAGE TEST

Start with half of a serving and wait 4 hours to fully assess your reaction to its strength and effects.

24 pitted prunes
1 cup orange juice
1 cup water
4 teaspoons canna-oil (page 105)
2 tablespoons brown sugar
½ teaspoon ground cinnamon

1. In a medium saucepan, combine the prunes, orange juice, water, canna-oil, brown sugar, and cinnamon.

2. Bring the mixture to a boil and immediately lower the heat, cover, and simmer gently for 25 to 30 minutes.

3. If there is too much liquid or if a thicker consistency is desired, remove the cover and simmer until the liquid is reduced.

4. Serve warm or chilled.

5. Store the remaining servings in an airtight container in the refrigerator for up to 4 days. Reheat in a small saucepan over low heat until warm, or enjoy chilled.

- -

You can swap out half of the prunes for dried apricots, another great source of fiber, potassium, iron, and antioxidants.

PER SERVING Calories: 144; Total Fat: 5.8g; Saturated Fat: 4.2g; Cholesterol: 0mg; Carbohydrates: 204.3g; Fiber: 21.7g; Protein: 7g

ROASTED BANANA PUDDING

GLUTEN-FREE | NUT-FREE | SOY-FREE | VEGETARIAN

Roasted bananas are amazingly sweet. A rich source of potassium and fiber, bananas are a naturally sweet treat packed with nutrients. When you add Greek yogurt, you also get a good dose of protein, probiotics, potassium, and calcium.

MAKES 2 SERVINGS

Prep time: 10 minutes
Cook time: 15 minutes

Required Equipment
Food processor or blender

 DOSAGE TEST

Start with half of a serving and wait 4 hours to fully assess your reaction to its strength and effects.

2 bananas, sliced
2 tablespoons honey
2 teaspoons canna-butter (page 106)
½ teaspoon ground cinnamon
⅔ cup vanilla Greek yogurt

1. Heat the oven to 340ºF.

2. Place the bananas on a rimmed baking sheet.

3. Drizzle the bananas with the honey, dot with the canna-butter, and sprinkle with the cinnamon.

4. Roast for 15 minutes. Remove from the oven and allow to cool.

5. In a food processor or blender, combine the bananas and yogurt. Blend for 1 to 2 minutes until smooth.

6. Serve immediately or chill in the refrigerator.

7. Store the remaining serving in an airtight container in the refrigerator for up to 3 days. Enjoy chilled.

- -

For a nice crunch, sprinkle a small handful of toasted coconut or pecan pieces on top of the pudding.

PER SERVING Calories: 277; Total Fat: 5.5g; Saturated Fat: 3.4g; Cholesterol: 18mg; Carbohydrates: 54.7g; Fiber: 3.4g; Protein: 7.4g

FIVE-INGREDIENT BANANA MUFFINS

GLUTEN-FREE | SOY-FREE | SUGAR-FREE | VEGETARIAN

You can enjoy this healthy muffin any time of day, but it is a great way to start your morning.

MAKES 12 MUFFINS

[1 muffin = 1 serving]
Prep time: 10 minutes
Cook time: 25 minutes

Required Equipment
Food processor

 DOSAGE TEST

Start with half of a serving and wait 4 hours to fully assess your reaction to its strength and effects.

3 very ripe bananas
3 large eggs
¾ cup peanut butter
¼ cup canna-oil (page 105)
¾ teaspoon baking powder

1. Preheat the oven to 340ºF.

2. In a food processor, combine the bananas, eggs, peanut butter, canna-oil, and baking powder. Process for 1 to 2 minutes until smooth.

3. Pour the mixture into a nonstick, or greased, muffin pan.

4. Bake for 20 to 25 minutes until golden brown and set.

5. Allow to cool before serving.

6. Store the remaining servings at room temperature in an airtight container for up to 3 days.

- -

If you don't mind adding a sixth ingredient, toss in a handful of chocolate chips before blending for chocolate muffins or after blending for chocolate-chip muffins.

PER SERVING Calories: 143; Total Fat: 9.5g; Saturated Fat: 2.1g; Cholesterol: 47mg; Carbohydrates: 11.2g; Fiber: 1.8g; Protein: 6g

PEANUT BUTTER AND BANANA SANDWICH

SOY-FREE | VEGAN

The crunch of the peanut butter and the chia seeds pairs wonderfully with the smooth texture of the banana in this delicious sandwich.

MAKES 1 SERVING

Prep time: 10 minutes

 DOSAGE TEST

Start with half of a serving and wait 4 hours to fully assess your reaction to its strength and effects.

½ banana, thinly sliced
1 teaspoon orange juice
3 tablespoons crunchy peanut butter
1 teaspoon agave
1 teaspoon canna-oil (page 105)
1 teaspoon chia seeds
Pinch ground cinnamon
2 slices whole-grain bread

1. In a small bowl, toss the banana slices with the orange juice.

2. In a separate small bowl, combine the peanut butter, agave, canna-oil, chia seeds, and cinnamon. Stir well.

3. Spread the peanut butter mixture evenly on 1 bread slice.

4. Top with the banana slices.

5. Close the sandwich with the remaining slice of bread.

6. Serve immediately or store in the refrigerator in an airtight container for up to 2 days.

- -

You can turn this sandwich into a gooey panini by grilling both sides in a skillet with a light coating of coconut oil until golden brown, about 4 minutes per side.

PER SERVING Calories: 504; Total Fat: 30.9g; Saturated Fat: 9.6g; Cholesterol: 0mg; Carbohydrates: 48.2g; Fiber: 8.6g; Protein: 18.7g

SLOW-COOKER APPLE-BERRY SAUCE

GLUTEN-FREE | NUT-FREE | SOY-FREE | SUGAR-FREE | VEGAN

It is quite possible that once you've made this recipe, you will never buy a jar of apple-sauce at the grocery store again. It is a refreshing and perfectly spiced sauce.

MAKES 9 SERVINGS

Prep time: 15 minutes
Cook time: 4 hours

Required Equipment
Slow cooker

 DOSAGE TEST

Start with half of a serving and wait 4 hours to fully assess your reaction to its strength and effects.

8 apples, peeled (if desired), cored, and sliced
1 (10-ounce) package frozen strawberries
2 tablespoons freshly squeezed lemon juice
3 tablespoons canna-oil (page 105)
1 teaspoon ground cinnamon
¼ teaspoon ground nutmeg

1. In a slow cooker, arrange the apple slices evenly on the bottom, and then add the remaining ingredients.

2. Cook on high for 4 hours until the apples are tender.

3. Enjoy warm or chill before serving.

4. Store the remaining servings in an airtight container in the refrigerator for up to 10 days.

- -

If the apples and berries aren't particularly sweet, you may want to add honey or agave to the sauce. Taste the sauce when approaching completion, and if it is not sweet enough to suit your taste, add a teaspoon of sweetener at a time to reach the desired sweetness.

PER SERVING Calories: 78; Total Fat: 0.3g; Saturated Fat: 0g; Cholesterol: 0mg; Carbohydrates: 20.6g; Fiber: 3.7g; Protein: 0.4g

DATE AND ALMOND SMOOTHIE

GLUTEN-FREE | SOY-FREE | SUGAR-FREE | VEGAN

This is a great smoothie for breakfast or an afternoon pick-me-up. It's also easy to prepare, so if you're hungry, you won't have to fuss much before enjoying this satisfying beverage.

MAKES 1 SERVING

Prep time: 10 minutes

Required Equipment
Blender

 DOSAGE TEST

Start with half of a serving and wait 4 hours to fully assess your reaction to its strength and effects.

1½ cups almond milk
½ small ripe banana, sliced
4 pitted dates
2 tablespoons almond butter
1 teaspoon canna-oil (page 105)
½ teaspoon ground cinnamon

1. In a blender, combine all the ingredients.

2. Pulse a few times and then blend on high speed for 1 to 2 minutes until smooth.

3. Serve immediately.

- -

Whenever you make a smoothie, it is usually a good idea to pour the liquid ingredients into the blender first.

PER SERVING Calories: 444; Total Fat: 28.2 g; Saturated Fat: 6.1g; Cholesterol: 0mg; Carbohydrates: 46g; Fiber: 7.3g; Protein: 9.7g

THREE-BERRY AND CHIA SEED SMOOTHIE

GLUTEN-FREE | SOY-FREE | VEGETARIAN

Raspberries, strawberries, and blueberries are packed with antioxidants. If you can't get fresh berries, frozen berries are a good alternative. This smoothie is delicious either way.

MAKES 1 SERVING

Prep time: 10 minutes

Required Equipment
Blender

 DOSAGE TEST

Start with half of a serving and wait 4 hours to fully assess your reaction to its strength and effects.

1 cup almond milk
½ cup plain yogurt
1 teaspoon canna-oil (page 105)
½ frozen banana, sliced
½ cup fresh raspberries
½ cup fresh strawberries
¼ cup fresh blueberries
1 tablespoon chia seeds
1 tablespoon honey

1. In a blender, combine all the ingredients.

2. Pulse a few times and then blend on high speed for 1 to 2 minutes until smooth.

3. Serve immediately.

- -

Add some cocoa powder or matcha (powdered green tea) for a flavorful antioxidant boost. For a creamier texture, you can add a little more yogurt.

PER SERVING Calories: 273; Total Fat: 11.1g; Saturated Fat: 4.5g; Cholesterol: 0mg; Carbohydrates: 47.7g; Fiber: 8g; Protein: 4.1g

CARAMEL BANANAS
WITH VANILLA YOGURT

GLUTEN-FREE | NUT-FREE | SOY-FREE | VEGETARIAN

Bananas are a versatile fruit. When frozen, they are creamy, like nature's ice cream. When raw, they are satisfying and simple. Caramelized bananas are smoky, sweet, and rich. Caramelizing them may become your favorite way to prepare bananas.

MAKES 2 SERVINGS
Prep time: 5 minutes
Cook time: 10 minutes

 DOSAGE TEST

Start with half of a serving and wait 4 hours to fully assess your reaction to its strength and effects.

1 tablespoon butter
2 teaspoons canna-butter (page 106)
2 tablespoons maple syrup
1 large banana, sliced
⅔ cup vanilla yogurt

1. In a small sauté pan or skillet, melt the butters. Add the maple syrup, and stir to combine.

2. Add the banana slices, and stir to coat. Cook for 7 to 9 minutes until the banana has begun to soften.

3. Divide the yogurt between 2 bowls. Add equal amounts of the caramelized bananas on top.

4. Serve while the bananas are warm.

5. Cover the remaining serving with plastic wrap and store in the refrigerator for up to 2 days. Enjoy chilled.

- -

If the bananas are very ripe, they will fall apart during the cooking. The taste will remain the same, but something may be lost in the presentation.

PER SERVING Calories: 197; Total Fat: 9.8g; Saturated Fat: 6.2g; Cholesterol: 25mg; Carbohydrates: 28.9g; Fiber: 1.8g; Protein: 0.8g

DARK CHOCOLATE DIPPED MANGO

GLUTEN-FREE | NUT-FREE | SOY-FREE | VEGETARIAN

The beauty of using dried fruit in this dessert is that it will last longer than fresh fruit. Plus, the chewiness of the fruit goes great with the smooth chocolate.

MAKES 6 SLICES

[3 slices = 1 serving]
Prep time: 15 minutes,
   plus 30 minutes setting time
Cook time: 10 minutes

Required Equipment
Double boiler

 DOSAGE TEST

Start with half of a serving and wait 4 hours to fully assess your reaction to its strength and effects.

½ cup dark chocolate chips or melting wafers
2 teaspoons canna-oil (page 105)
6 pieces dried mango

1. Prepare your work surface by spreading out a piece of parchment paper or aluminum foil.

2. In a double boiler, combine the chocolate and canna-oil. Heat over medium heat, stirring as needed, until fully melted. Remove from the heat.

3. Dip the mango pieces in the melted chocolate one at a time and place on the parchment paper, spacing them evenly apart.

4. Allow to set for at least 30 minutes.

5. Store the slices in an airtight container at room temperature for up to 1 week or in the refrigerator for up to 2 weeks.

- -

If the chocolate gets too hot or water gets into the bowl, the chocolate can seize up and get lumpy, so be careful. You can substitute any type of dried fruit for the mango in this recipe.

PER SERVING Calories: 228; Total Fat: 25.2g; Saturated Fat: 15.0 g; Cholesterol: 0mg; Carbohydrates: 25.8g; Fiber: 6.9g; Protein: 3.4g

GRAHAM CRACKERS
WITH PEANUT BUTTER AND BANANA

SOY-FREE | SUGAR-FREE | VEGAN

Whether you use the creamy or crunchy type, peanut butter pairs well with bananas. Spread it on top of graham crackers, and you have a yummy treat that makes a great breakfast, snack, or dessert.

MAKES 2 SERVINGS
Prep time: 10 minutes

 DOSAGE TEST

Start with half of a serving and wait 4 hours to fully assess your reaction to its strength and effects.

2 double graham crackers
1 banana, sliced
1 teaspoon freshly squeezed lemon juice
6 tablespoons peanut butter
2 teaspoons canna-oil (page 105)
2 tablespoons shredded unsweetened coconut

1. Place the graham crackers on your work surface.

2. In a small bowl, toss the banana slices with the lemon juice.

3. In a separate bowl, combine the peanut butter and canna-oil. Stir well to combine.

4. Spread half of the peanut butter mixture on each graham cracker.

5. Top each cracker with an equal portion of the sliced banana.

6. Sprinkle with the coconut.

7. Serve.

8. Store the remaining serving in an airtight container in the refrigerator for up to 3 days.

- -

To make a frozen treat out of this recipe, mash the banana and mix it with the peanut butter before spreading it on the graham crackers. Top it off with an additional graham cracker and pop it in the freezer for a few hours. (If you like hazelnut chocolate spread, you can swap it for the peanut butter in either method.)

PER SERVING Calories: 322; Total Fat: 26g; Saturated Fat: 6.7g; Cholesterol: 0mg; Carbohydrates: 23.7g; Fiber: 4.8g; Protein: 12g

MEDICAL MARIJUANA LAWS BY STATE

The information in these tables was last updated January 2016. For the most up-to-date information on marijuana laws in your state, please visit norml.org/laws.

RECREATIONAL STATES

In the states listed in the following table, adults can consume cannabis without facing legal action if they adhere to the outlined requirements. These states also have medical marijuana programs, details of which you can find in the table on page 192.

Possession Limit	Cultivation	Notes
ALASKA		
1 ounce	6 plants (3 mature, 3 immature)	For more information, visit dhss.alaska.gov/dph /Director/Pages/marijuana/law.aspx.
COLORADO		
1 ounce	6 plants (3 mature, 3 immature)	For more information, visit www.colorado.gov /pacific/marijuanainfodenver/residents-visitors.
DISTRICT OF COLUMBIA (WASHINGTON, DC)		
2 ounces	6 plants (3 mature, 3 immature)	For more information, visit norml.org/laws/item /district-of-columbia-penalties.
OREGON		
8 ounces at home; 1 ounce in public	4 plants	For more information, visit www.oregon.gov /olcc/marijuana.
WASHINGTON		
1 ounce; 7 grams concentrate; 16 ounces edible in solid form; 72 ounces edible in liquid form	None	For more information, visit www.liq.wa.gov /mj2015/fact-sheet.

MEDICAL STATES

There are medical marijuana programs in 23 states and in the District of Columbia. The following table provides an overview of the possession and cultivation limits, along with approved conditions for obtaining a medical marijuana card. Each state has unique laws to govern their medical programs, so be sure you know what's allowed in your state. Follow the provided links for more information on each state's program and how to apply.

Possession Limit	Cultivation	Approved Conditions
ALASKA		
1 ounce	6 plants (3 mature, 3 immature)	Cachexia, cancer, chronic pain, epilepsy and other disorders characterized by seizures, glaucoma, HIV, AIDS, multiple sclerosis and other disorders characterized by muscle spasticity, and nausea. Other conditions are subject to approval by the Alaska Department of Health and Social Services. For more information, visit dhss.alaska.gov/dph/VitalStats/Pages/marijuana.aspx.
ARIZONA		
2.5 ounces	12 plants if the patient lives more than 25 miles from the nearest dispensary	Cancer, glaucoma, HIV, AIDS, hepatitis C, ALS, Crohn's disease, Alzheimer's disease, cachexia/wasting syndrome, severe and chronic pain, severe nausea, seizures (including epilepsy), severe or persistent muscle spasms (including multiple sclerosis), and PTSD. For more information, visit www.azdhs.gov/medicalmarijuana/index.htm.
CALIFORNIA		
8 ounces	6 mature or 12 immature plants	Anorexia, arthritis, cachexia, cancer, chronic pain, glaucoma, HIV, AIDS, migraines, persistent muscle spasms (including spasms associated with multiple sclerosis), seizures (including seizures associated with epilepsy), severe nausea, and other chronic or persistent medical symptoms. For more information, visit www.cdph.ca.gov/programs/mmp/Pages/default.aspx.
COLORADO		
1 ounce	6 plants (3 mature, 3 immature)	Cachexia, cancer, chronic pain, chronic nervous system disorders, glaucoma, HIV, AIDS, nausea, persistent muscle spasms, and seizures. For more information, visit www.colorado.gov/pacific/marijuanainfodenver/residents-visitors.

Possession Limit	Cultivation	Approved Conditions
CONNECTICUT		
1-month supply	None	Cancer, glaucoma, HIV, AIDS, Parkinson's disease, multiple sclerosis, damage to the nervous tissue of the spinal cord with objective neurological indication of intractable spasticity, epilepsy, cachexia or wasting syndrome, Crohn's disease, PTSD, or any other medical condition or disease approved by Connecticut's Department of Consumer Protection. For more information, visit www.ct.gov/dcp/cwp/view.asp?a=1620&q=503670.
DELAWARE		
6 ounces	None	Cancer, HIV, AIDS, hepatitis C, ALS, Alzheimer's disease, PTSD, and chronic or debilitating disease or medical condition or its treatment that produces one or more of the following: cachexia/wasting syndrome; severe, debilitating pain; intractable nausea; seizures; or severe and persistent muscle spasms, including but not limited to those characteristic of multiple sclerosis. For more information, visit dhss.delaware.gov/dhss/dph/hsp/medmarhome.html.
DISTRICT OF COLUMBIA		
2 ounces	None	HIV, AIDS, cancer, glaucoma, conditions characterized by severe and persistent muscle spasms such as multiple sclerosis, patients undergoing chemotherapy or radiotherapy, or patients using azidothymidine or protease inhibitors. For more information, visit doh.dc.gov/node/157882.
HAWAII		
4 ounces	7 plants	Cancer, glaucoma, HIV, AIDS, PTSD, chronic or debilitating disease or medical condition or its treatment that produces cachexia/wasting syndrome, severe pain, severe nausea, seizures (including those characteristic of epilepsy), or severe and persistent muscle spasms (including those characteristic of multiple sclerosis or Crohn's disease). Other conditions are subject to approval by the Hawaii Department of Health. For more information, visit health.hawaii.gov/medicalmarijuana/.

Possession Limit	Cultivation	Approved Conditions
ILLINOIS		
2.5 ounces	None	Cancer, glaucoma, HIV, AIDS, hepatitis C, ALS, Crohn's disease, agitation of Alzheimer's disease, cachexia/wasting syndrome, muscular dystrophy, severe fibromyalgia, spinal cord disease (including but not limited to arachnoiditis), Tarlov cysts, hydromyelia, syringomyelia, rheumatoid arthritis, fibrous dysplasia, spinal cord injury, traumatic brain injury and post-concussion syndrome, multiple sclerosis, Arnold–Chiari malformation, spinocerebellar ataxia (SCA), Parkinson's disease, Tourette syndrome, myoclonus, dystonia, reflex sympathetic dystrophy (RSD), causalgia, complex regional pain syndrome type II (CRPS), neurofibromatosis, chronic inflammatory demyelinating polyneuropathy, chronic inflammatory demyelinating polyneuropathy, Sjögren's syndrome, lupus, interstitial cystitis, myasthenia gravis, hydrocephalus, nail–patella syndrome or residual limb pain, and seizures (including those related to epilepsy). For more information, visit www.idph.state.il.us/HealthWellness/MedicalCannabis/index.htm.
MAINE		
2.5 ounces	6 mature plants	Cancer, HIV, AIDS, hepatitis C, ALS, Crohn's disease, epilepsy and other disorders characterized by seizures, glaucoma, multiple sclerosis and other disorders characterized by muscle spasticity, nail–patella syndrome, chronic intractable pain, cachexia/wasting syndrome, and severe nausea. For more information, visit www.maine.gov/dhhs/dlrs/mmm/index.shtml.
MARYLAND		
4 ounces	None	Cachexia/wasting syndrome, anorexia, severe or chronic pain, severe nausea, seizures, severe or persistent muscle spasms, or other conditions approved by Maryland's Medical Marijuana Commission. For more information on Maryland's medical marijuana program, visit mmcc.maryland.gov/.
MASSACHUSETTS		
60-day supply (10 ounces marijuana or 1.5 ounces concentrate)	Allowed in limited amounts for 60-day supply	Cancer, glaucoma, positive status for HIV or AIDS, hepatitis C, ALS, Crohn's disease, Parkinson's disease, multiple sclerosis, and other conditions as determined in writing by a qualifying patient's physician. For more information, visit www.mass.gov/medicalmarijuana.

Possession Limit	Cultivation	Approved Conditions
MICHIGAN		
2.5 ounces	12 plants	Cancer, glaucoma, HIV, AIDS, hepatitis C, ALS, Crohn's disease, agitation of Alzheimer's disease, nail–patella syndrome, cachexia, severe and chronic pain, severe nausea, seizures, epilepsy, muscle spasms, multiple sclerosis, and PTSD. For more information, visit www.michigan.gov/mmp.
MINNESOTA		
1.5 ounces	None	Cancer associated with severe/chronic pain, nausea or severe vomiting, or cachexia or severe wasting; glaucoma; HIV/AIDS; Tourette syndrome; ALS; seizures, including those characteristic of epilepsy; severe and persistent muscle spasms, including those characteristic of multiple sclerosis; Crohn's disease; terminal illness, with a probable life expectancy of less than one year. For more information, visit www.health.state.mn.us/topics/cannabis.
MONTANA		
1 ounce	16 plants (4 mature, 12 immature)	Cancer, glaucoma, or positive status for HIV or AIDS when the condition or disease results in symptoms that seriously and adversely affect the patient's health status, cachexia/wasting syndrome, severe and chronic pain that significantly interferes with daily activities as documented by the patient's treating physician, intractable nausea or vomiting, epilepsy or intractable seizure disorder, multiple sclerosis, Crohn's disease, painful peripheral neuropathy, central nervous system disorder resulting in chronic and painful spasticity or muscle spasms, and admittance into hospice care. For more information, visit dphhs.mt.gov/marijuana.
NEVADA		
2.5 ounces	12 plants	AIDS; cancer; glaucoma; any medical condition or treatment to a medical condition that produces cachexia, persistent muscle spasms or seizures, or severe nausea or pain; and PTSD. Other conditions are subject to approval by the Nevada Division of Public and Behavioral Health. For more information, visit dpbh.nv.gov/Reg/Medical_Marijuana/.

Possession Limit	Cultivation	Approved Conditions
NEW HAMPSHIRE		
2 ounces	None	Cancer, glaucoma, HIV, AIDS, hepatitis C, ALS, muscular dystrophy, Crohn's disease, agitation of Alzheimer's disease, multiple sclerosis, chronic pancreatitis, spinal cord injury or disease, traumatic brain injury, seizures, severe and persistent muscle spasms, or a severely debilitating or terminal medical condition or its treatment that produces elevated intraocular pressure, cachexia/wasting syndrome, chemotherapy-induced anorexia, or severe pain. For more information, visit www.dhhs.state.nh.us/oos/tcp/index.htm.
NEW JERSEY		
2 ounces during a 30-day period	None	Seizure disorder, epilepsy, intractable skeletal muscular spasticity, glaucoma, severe or chronic pain, severe nausea or vomiting, cachexia, HIV, AIDS, ALS, multiple sclerosis, terminal cancer, muscular dystrophy, inflammatory bowel disease, Crohn's disease, terminal illness, or any other medical condition or its treatment that is approved by New Jersey's Department of Health and Senior Services. For more information, visit www.state.nj.us/health/med_marijuana.shtml.
NEW MEXICO		
6 ounces	16 plants (4 mature, 12 immature)	Severe chronic pain, painful peripheral neuropathy, intractable nausea/vomiting, severe anorexia, cachexia, hepatitis C infection, Crohn's disease, PTSD, ALS, cancer, glaucoma, multiple sclerosis, damage to the nervous tissue of the spinal cord with intractable spasticity, epilepsy, HIV, AIDS, hospice patients, cervical dystonia, inflammatory autoimmune-mediated arthritis, Parkinson's disease, and Huntington's disease. For more information, visit nmhealth.org/about/mcp/svcs/.
NEW YORK		
30-day supply; only non-smokable cannabis products	None	Cancer, HIV, AIDS, ALS, Parkinson's disease, multiple sclerosis, spinal cord injury with spasticity, epilepsy, inflammatory bowel disease, neuropathy, and Huntington's disease. Associated or complicating conditions: cachexia/wasting syndrome, severe or chronic pain, severe nausea, seizures, or severe or persistent muscle spasms. For more information, visit www.health.ny.gov/regulations/medical_marijuana/faq.htm.

Possession Limit	Cultivation	Approved Conditions
OREGON		
24 ounces	24 plants (6 mature, 18 immature)	Cancer; glaucoma; positive status for HIV or AIDS or treatment for these conditions; a medical condition or treatment for a medical condition that produces cachexia, severe pain, or severe nausea; seizures (including seizures caused by epilepsy); or persistent muscle spasms (including spasms caused by multiple sclerosis). Other conditions are subject to approval by the Health Division of the Oregon Department of Human Resources. For more information, visit www.oregon.gov/oha/mmj/Pages/index.aspx.
RHODE ISLAND		
2.5 ounces	24 plants (12 mature, 12 immature)	Cancer, glaucoma, positive status for HIV or AIDS, hepatitis C, or the treatment of these conditions; a chronic or debilitating disease or medical condition or its treatment that produces cachexia/wasting syndrome; severe, debilitating, chronic pain; severe nausea; seizures, including but not limited to those characteristic of epilepsy; severe and persistent muscle spasms, including but not limited to those characteristic of multiple sclerosis or Crohn's disease; agitation of Alzheimer's disease; or any other medical condition or its treatment approved by the state Department of Health. For more information, visit www.health.ri.gov/healthcare/medicalmarijuana/index.php.
VERMONT		
2 ounces	9 plants (2 mature, 7 immature)	Cancer, AIDS, positive status for HIV, multiple sclerosis, or the treatment of these conditions if the disease or the treatment results in severe, persistent, and intractable symptoms; or a disease, medical condition, or its treatment that is chronic, debilitating, and produces severe, persistent, and one or more of the following intractable symptoms: cachexia/wasting syndrome, severe pain, or nausea or seizures. For more information, visit vcic.vermont.gov/marijuana-registry.
WASHINGTON		
3 ounces; 21 grams concentrate; 48 ounces edible in solid form; 216 ounces edible in liquid form	6–15 mature plants, depending on medical need	Cachexia, cancer, Crohn's disease, glaucoma, hepatitis C, HIV, AIDS, intractable pain, persistent muscle spasms and/or spasticity, nausea, PTSD, seizures, traumatic brain injury, or any "terminal or debilitating condition." For more information, visit www.liq.wa.gov/mj2015/fact-sheet.

ILLEGAL STATES

While many states have legislation underway, there are 27 states that have no true medical marijuana programs at the time of this writing. Some of them have permitted CBD oil for medical purposes, which is a great first step, but it still falls short. If you live in one of the following states and choose to pursue the medicinal use of cannabis, it is important to be aware of the laws and risks involved.

Offense for Possession	Offense for Cultivation	Offense for Sale	Notes
ALABAMA Misdemeanor for first offense; felony for further possession or intent to sell	Felony	Felony	CBD oil is allowed for treating seizures and epilepsy.
ARKANSAS Misdemeanor under 4 ounces (113 grams)	Felony	Felony	
FLORIDA Misdemeanor under 20 grams	Felony	Misdemeanor under 20 grams	CBD oil is allowed for treating seizures and epilepsy.
GEORGIA Misdemeanor under 1 ounce (28 grams)	Felony	Felony	CBD oil is allowed for treating seizures and epilepsy.
IDAHO Misdemeanor under 3 ounces (84 grams)	Felony	Felony	
INDIANA Misdemeanor	Felony	Misdemeanor under 30 grams	
IOWA Misdemeanor	Felony	Felony	
KANSAS Misdemeanor (first offense)	Felony	Felony	
KENTUCKY Misdemeanor under 8 ounces (224 grams)	Misdemeanor under 5 plants	Misdemeanor under 8 ounces (224 grams)	CBD oil is allowed for treating seizures and epilepsy.

Offense for Possession	Offense for Cultivation	Offense for Sale	Notes
LOUISIANA 15-day incarceration for 14 grams or less (first offense)	Felony	Felony	The third possession offense is considered a felony.
MISSISSIPPI Decriminalized at 30 grams or less	Felony	Felony	CBD oil is allowed for treating seizures and epilepsy.
MISSOURI Misdemeanor under 35 grams	Felony	Felony	CBD oil is allowed for treating seizures and epilepsy. Decriminalization law takes effect January 1, 2017.
NEBRASKA Decriminalized up to 28 grams	Felony	Felony	Possession of up to 28 grams is treated as a civil infraction for the first offense, and as a misdemeanor for the second and third offenses (up to 1 pound).
NORTH CAROLINA Misdemeanor up to 1.5 ounces (42 grams)	Felony	Felony	CBD oil is allowed for treating seizures and epilepsy.
NORTH DAKOTA Misdemeanor up to 1 ounce (28 grams)	Felony	Felony	
OHIO Misdemeanor up to 200 grams	Felony	Misdemeanor for a gift up to 20 grams; felony for a sale of any amount	
OKLAHOMA Felony for second offense	Felony	Felony	CBD oil is allowed for children with epilepsy.

Offense for Possession	Offense for Cultivation	Offense for Sale	Notes
PENNSYLVANIA			
Misdemeanor	Felony	Misdemeanor up to 30 grams	Philadelphia has decriminalized up to 28 grams.
SOUTH CAROLINA			
Misdemeanor up to 1 ounce (28 grams)	Felony	Felony	CBD oil is allowed for treating seizures and epilepsy.
SOUTH DAKOTA			
Misdemeanor up to 2 ounces (56 grams)	Felony	Misdemeanor up to 14 grams	
TENNESSEE			
Misdemeanor up to 14 grams	Felony	Felony	The third offense for possession of up to 14 grams is a felony. CBD oil is allowed for treating seizures and epilepsy.
TEXAS			
Misdemeanor up to 4 ounces (113 grams)	Felony	Misdemeanor up to 7 grams	Low-THC, high-CBD cannabis is allowed for patients with intractable epilepsy.
UTAH			
Misdemeanor under 1 pound (453 grams)	Felony	Felony	CBD oil is allowed for treating severe, debilitating epileptic conditions.
VIRGINIA			
Misdemeanor	Felony	Felony	
WEST VIRGINIA			
Misdemeanor	Felony	Felony	
WISCONSIN			
Misdemeanor (first offense)	Felony	Felony	CBD oil is allowed for treating severe, debilitating epileptic conditions.
WYOMING			
Misdemeanor under 3 ounces (84 grams)	Misdemeanor	Felony	CBD oil is allowed for treating severe, debilitating epileptic conditions.

TEN TIPS FOR CULTIVATING CANNABIS AT HOME

With just a few tools and some patience, you can grow your own cannabis right at home. If you live in a state that does not legally allow cannabis cultivation at home, please understand the risks involved. Many states consider this a felony and will prosecute it as such. Refer to the table on page 198 to check the penalties in your state.

For those living in states allowing at-home cultivation, you are in luck! Growing can be a pleasant, stress-relieving activity on its own, and you can save money by growing your own medicine. Although growing cannabis can be relatively easy, it's not for everyone. Here are a few tips that can help get you started.

1. Ask for advice. If you know a grower, consult with them and ask them to walk you through the process. It helps to have a friend who has been through the process to advise and provide seasoned guidance.

2. Use a clone. If you have access, start with a clone (cuttings from a "mother" cannabis plant) from a reputable grower. If you can't get a clone, your best bet is to get a seed from a grower whose plant you enjoyed. Otherwise, purchase a seed from your local dispensary.

3. Keep only female plants. Unless your goal is producing seeds, remove any male plants that develop. They will not produce the beautiful buds you are looking for, and if they are in a room with female plants, they will cause the females to devote their energy to seed production and reduce overall potency.

4. Give your plant room to grow. Ensure your cannabis plant is in a container large enough to accommodate it. A pot with a 3-gallon capacity should do the trick.

5. Keep the environment warm and well lit. Cannabis is happiest at temperatures between 65°F and 80°F with 12 or more hours of sunlight. Don't grow outdoors unless your climate meets these conditions.

6. If growing indoors, set up a small, well-ventilated area and mount an LED grow light above your plant. It can help to have a small fan to circulate the air. Light the plant for 18 hours on, then 6 hours off for the first 4 weeks. Then transition to 12 hours on, 12 hours off to initiate the "flowering" stage. It will be another 2 to 3 months before your plant is ready.

7. Prepare a nurturing environment. Cannabis plants need plenty water. The rule of thumb is to water when the soil is dry—about once a week for young plants, once a day for mature plants. They need good soil with a pH close to 6.0 or 7.0, and special nutrients. If your leaves begin to yellow, you need to add fertilizer. If they develop ugly spots on the leaves, you may be giving it too much fertilizer.

8. Watch out for pests. Little white spots on the leaves of your plant may be a sign of spider mites, a common pest among cannabis plants. The best way to treat your plant is to spray it with neem oil during the dark hours.

9. Harvest when the plant tells you it's ready. When the pistils (the hair-like parts on the bud) darken and begin to curl, it is time to harvest your plant. Cut off all the branches, remove the fan leaves, trim the large sugar leaves (the leaves close to the buds that are covered in some amount of resin), and hang them upside down to dry. You could also dry them in a mesh drying rack.

10. Once your buds are completely dry (about a week), clip them from the branches and allow them to cure in closed, glass jars. Open the jars at least once a day for the first 2 weeks, then every couple of days for 2 weeks after that.

GLOSSARY

baked: The state of being very high from cannabis.

blunt: Cannabis wrapped in tobacco leaves from cigar wrappers and smoked like a joint.

bong: A water pipe that is used to smoke marijuana. Bongs can vary in shape and materials, but generally include a small bowl for the cannabis, a carburetor, and a large chamber containing water where the smoke collects before being inhaled.

bowl: The part of the pipe or bong where the cannabis is placed.

buds: The dried flowers of the cannabis plant. They contain the highest concentration of plant resin.

budtender: A "bartender" for weed. These are the people you will deal with when visiting a dispensary.

cannabidiol (CBD): A nonpsychoactive cannabinoid with a wide scope of potential health benefits.

cannabinoid: Naturally occurring chemical compounds found in the cannabis plant.

carb or carburetor: A hole in a bong or pipe. It is blocked when you draw smoke from the burning cannabis, and then released when you inhale the smoke into your lungs.

clone: A rooted clipping from a marijuana plant that allows you to plant the exact genetic match of the mother plant.

concentrate: An extraction with concentrated levels of cannabinoids. It can be in the form of oil, wax, shatter, or hash.

crystals: Another word for excreted resin on the cannabis flowers.

dab: A relatively new method of inhaling concentrated cannabis that produces an extremely potent vapor.

dank: Slang for strong-smelling, high-quality marijuana.

decarboxylate: The process of heating cannabis at a low temperature to transform THCA into the psychoactive compound THC.

dispensary: A licensed store selling cannabis and cannabis products.

edibles: Foods and drinks made with cannabis.

extraction: The process of stripping the cannabis plant of its important compounds to create a concentrate with more potent levels of the plant's cannabinoids.

ganja: A term for cannabis that originated from Rastafarians.

grinder: The device that breaks up cannabis buds into small, uniform granulates for smoking or vaping.

hash: Concentrated cannabis resin.

hemp: Cannabis that has very low THC and is used for industrial purposes.

hybrid: A strain of cannabis bred from an *indica* and a *sativa*.

indica: A species of cannabis that is known for producing a relaxing and restful high, as well as helping ease muscle pain, inflammation, and insomnia.

indoor: Cannabis that has been grown inside, requiring special equipment that includes lights to replicate the sun. Growing indoors allows for greater control of the plant.

joint: A rolled cigarette that is filled with cannabis.

kief: Dried resin from the cannabis plant.

munchies: The increased appetite caused by inhaling or ingesting cannabis.

oil/hash oil/cannabis oil: Dark, gooey concentrated oil typically found in plastic syringes. Made from solvents such as butane, ethanol, CO_2, isopropyl alcohol, or hexane.

outdoor: Cannabis grown outside with sunlight.

resin: The sticky, crystal-like matter containing cannabinoids and terpenes that is excreted from the cannabis plant, with the highest concentrations in the flower (bud).

sativa: A species of cannabis that is known for producing a euphoric and energizing high.

shake: Small pieces of bud, usually left after trimming the buds or collecting at the bottom of a jar or bag. Shake may also contain sugar leaves. It will still contain important compounds, although the potency may be weaker than pure bud depending on the quantity of leaves in the shake.

shatter: A very potent cannabis concentrate with varying levels of transparency. It is solid at cold temperatures.

strain: A genetic variant or subtype in the cannabis family that is created by breeding two distinct strains.

terpene: Compounds that give the different cannabis strains their unique flavor and smell. Terpenes are found in a variety of plants, not just cannabis.

tetrahydrocannabinol (THC): The most prevalent cannabinoid in marijuana, responsible for the psychoactive effects of the plant, as well as many health benefits.

tincture: A cannabis extract in liquid form, usually made with alcohol or vegetable glycerin.

topical: A cannabis-infused mixture used on the skin, such as a salve, lotion, or bath soak.

trichome: The glands of the cannabis plant that produce resin.

vape pen: A small, portable vaporizing device that holds either bud or cannabis concentrate.

vaporizer: A machine that turns flower or concentrates into vapor.

wax: A cannabis concentrate that is soft and opaque.

RESOURCES

BOOKS

Social/Political/Historical

David Bearman, *Drugs are NOT the Devil's Tools: How Discrimination and Greed Created a Dysfunctional Drug Policy and How It Can Be Fixed*, Blue Point Books, 2014.

Richard J. Bonnie and Charles H. Whitebread, *The Marijuana Conviction: A History of Marijuana Prohibition in the United States*, The Lindesmith Center, 1999.

Steve DeAngelo, *The Cannabis Manifesto: A New Paradigm for Wellness*, North Atlantic Books, 2015.

Steve Fox, Paul Armentano, and Mason Tvert, *Marijuana Is Safer: So Why Are We Driving People to Drink?*, 2nd edition, Chelsea Green, 2013.

Jack Herer, *The Emperor Wears No Clothes: Hemp and the Marijuana Conspiracy*, 12th edition, Ah Ha Publishing, 2010.

Julie Holland (ed.), *The Pot Book*, Park Street Press, 2010.

Martin A. Lee, *Smoke Signals: A Social History of Marijuana—Medical, Recreational, and Scientific*, Scribner, 2012.

Medical

Michael Backes, *Cannabis Pharmacy: The Practical Guide to Medical Marijuana*, Black Dog & Leventhal, 2014.

David Casarett, *Stoned: A Doctor's Case for Medical Marijuana*, Current, 2015.

John Hicks, *The Medicinal Power of Cannabis: Using a Natural Herb to Heal Arthritis, Nausea, Pain, and Other Ailments*, Skyhorse Publishing, 2015.

Ed Rosenthal, *Beyond Buds: Marijuana Extracts—Hash, Vaping, Dabbing, Edibles, and Medicines*, Quick American Archives, 2014.

Clint Werner, *Marijuana Gateway to Health: How Cannabis Protects Us from Cancer and Alzheimer's Disease*, Dachstar Press, 2011.

Growing

Jorges Cervantes, *Marijuana Grow Basics: The Easy Guide for Cannabis Aficionados*, Van Patten Publishing, 2009.

Greg Green, *The Cannabis Grow Bible: The Definitive Guide to Growing Marijuana for Recreational and Medical Use*, 2nd edition, Green Candy Press, 2009.

Ed Rosenthal, *Marijuana Grower's Handbook: Your Complete Guide for Medical and Personal Marijuana Cultivation*, Quick American Archives, 2010.

WEBSITES & ORGANIZATIONS

NORML.org
National Organization for the Reform of
Marijuana Laws

Lawyers.norml.org
Find a lawyer and member of NORML's legal
committee

Cancer.gov/about-cancer/treatment/cam
/patient/cannabis-pdq
The National Cancer Institute's knowledge
base on cannabis and cannabinoids in cancer
treatments

CannabisCulture.com
Cannabis culture and news

CannabisHealth.com
Global resource for the health and science
of cannabis

TheCannabist.co
News, reviews, and recipes from the Denver
Post's marijuana section

DrugPolicy.org
Drug Policy Alliance

ENCOD.org
European Coalition for Just and Effective
Drug Policy (ENCOD)

HighTimes.com
Marijuana news and culture

Leafly.com
Marijuana dispensary and strain reviews

Leafly.com/doctors
Find a doctor in states with medical marijuana laws

LeafScience.com
Marijuana news, facts, and medical research

LetFreedomGrow.com
The American Alliance for Medical Cannabis

MPP.org
Marijuana Policy Project

SafeAccessNow.org
Americans for Safe Access

Verdabase.com
Knowledge base of cannabis strains

VeteransForMedicalMarijuana.org
Veterans for Medical Cannabis Access

WomenGrow.com
Women Grow

REFERENCES

Abrams, D. I., C. A. Jay, S. B. Shade, H. Vizoso, H. Reda, S. Press, M. E. Kelly, M. C. Rowbotham, and K. L. Petersen. "Cannabis in Painful HIV-Associated Sensory Neuropathy: A Randomized Placebo-Controlled Trial." *Neurology* 68, no. 7 (February 2007): 515–21, www.ncbi.nlm.nih.gov/pubmed/17296917.

Alshaarway, O., and J. C. Anthony. "Cannabis Smoking and Diabetes Mellitus: Results from Meta-Analysis with Eight Independent Replication Samples." *Epidemiology* 26, no. 4 (July 2015): 597–600. doi:10.1097/EDE.0000000000000314.

American Academy of Neurology. "Medical Marijuana Liquid Extract May Bring Hope for Children with Severe Epilepsy." April 13, 2015. www.aan.com/PressRoom/home/PressRelease/1364.

Amtmann, D., P. Weydt, K. L. Johnson, M. P. Jensen, and G. T. Carter. "Survey of Cannabis Use in Patients with Amyotrophic Lateral Sclerosis." *American Journal of Hospice and Palliative Care* 21, no. 2 (March–April 2004): 95–104, www.ncbi.nlm.nih.gov/pubmed/15055508.

Appendino, Giovanni, Simon Gibbons, Anna Giana, Alberto Pagani, Gianpaolo Grassi, Michael Stavri, Eileen Smith, and M. Mukhlesur Rahman. "Antibacterial Cannabinoids from Cannabis Sativa: A Structure Study." *Journal of Natural Products* 71, no. 8 (August 2008): 1427–30. doi:10.1021/np8002673.

Bab, I., A. Zimmer, and E. Melamed. "Cannabinoids and the Skeleton: From Marijuana to Reversal of Bone Loss." *Annals of Medicine* 41, no. 8 (2009): 560–67. doi:10.1080/07853890903121025.

Bachhuber, Marcus A. "Medical Cannabis Laws and Opioid Analgesic Overdose Mortality in the United States, 1999–2010." *JAMA Internal Medicine* 174, no. 10 (2014): 1668–73. doi:10.1001/jamainternmed.2014.4005.

BBC News. "Cannabis Lifts Alzheimer's Appetite." August 21, 2003. news.bbc.co.uk/2/hi/health/3169901.stm.

Ben-Shabat, Shimon. "An Entourage Effect: Inactive Endogenous Fatty Acid Glycerol Esters Enhance 2-arachidonoyl-glycerol Cannabinoid Activity." *European Journal of Pharmacology* 353, no. 1 (July 1998): 23–31.

Bernstein, David. "Hepatitis C—Current State of the Art and Future Directions." *MedScape Today.* December 8, 2004. www.medscape.org/viewarticle/495211.

Blake, D. R., P. Robson, M. Ho, R. W. Jubb, and C. S. McCabe. "Preliminary Assessment of the Efficacy, Tolerability and Safety of a Cannabis Medicine (Sativex) in the Treatment of Pain Caused by Rheumatoid Arthritis." *Rheumatology* 45, no. 1 (January 2006): 50–52. www.ncbi.nlm.nih.gov/pubmed/16282192.

Borrelli, F., I. Fasolino, B. Romano, R. Capasso, F. Maiello, D. Coppola, P. Orlando, et al. "Beneficial Effect of the Non-Psychotropic Plant Cannabinoid Cannabigerol on Experimental Inflammatory Bowel Disease." *Biochemical Pharmacology* 85, no. 9 (May 2013): 1306–16. doi:10.1016/j.bcp.2013.01.017.

Boychuk, D. G., G. Goddard, G. Mauro, and M. F. Orellana. "The Effectiveness of Cannabinoids in the Management of Chronic Nonmalignant Neuropathic Pain: A Systematic Review." *Journal of Oral & Facial Pain and Headache* 29, no. 1 (2015): 7–14. doi:10.11607/ofph.1274.

Brenneisen, R., A. Egli, M. A. Elsohly, V. Henn, and Y. Spiess. "The Effect of Orally and Rectally Administered Delta 9-Tetrahydrocannabinol on Spasticity: A Pilot Study with 2 Patients." *International Journal of Clinical Pharmacology and Therapeutics* 34, no. 10 (October 1996): 446–52. www.ncbi.nlm.nih.gov/pubmed/8897084.

Brown, David T. *Cannabis: The Genius Plant*. Amsterdam, The Netherlands: Harwood Academic Publishers, 2003.

Carley, D. W., S. Paviovic, M. Janelidze, and M. Radulovacki. "Functional Role for Cannabinoids in Respiratory Stability During Sleep." *Sleep* 25, no. 4 (June 2002): 391–98. www.ncbi.nlm.nih.gov/pubmed/12071539.

Centers for Disease Control and Prevention. "National Vital Statistics System: Mortality Data." December 30, 2015. www.cdc.gov/nchs/deaths.htm.

Chagas, M. H., A. W. Zuardi, V. Tumas, M. A. Pena-Pereira, E. T. Sobreira, M. M.

Bergamaschi, A. C. dos Santos, et al. "Effects of Cannabidiol in the Treatment of Patients with Parkinson's Disease: An Exploratory Double-Blind Trial." *Journal of Psychopharmacology* 28, no. 11 (November 2014): 1088–98. doi:10.1177/0269881114550355.

Chatterjee, Avijit, Almahrezi, Ware, and Fitzcharles. "A Dramatic Response to Inhaled Cannabis in a Woman with Central Thalamic Pain and Dystonia." *The Journal of Pain and Symptom Management* 24, no. 1 (July 2002): 4–6, doi:10.1016/S0885-3924(02)00426-8.

CNN. "CNN Poll: Support for Legal Marijuana Soaring." January 6, 2014. politicalticker.blogs.cnn.com/2014/01/06/cnn-poll-support-for-legal-marijuana-soaring.

Cooper, Z. D., S. D. Comer, and M. Haney. "Comparison of the Analgesic Effects of Dronabinol and Smoked Marijuana in Daily Marijuana Smokers." *Neuropsychopharmacology* 38, no. 10 (September 2013): 1984–92. doi:10.1038/npp.2013.97.

Corey-Bloom, Jody. "Short-Term Effects of Cannabis Therapy on Spasticity in Multiple Sclerosis." In: University of San Diego Health Sciences, Center for Medicinal Cannabis Research. *Report to the Legislature and Governor of the State of California presenting findings pursuant to SB847 which created the CMCR and provided state funding*. 2010.

Di Carlo, G. and A. A. Izzo, "Cannabinoids for Gastrointestinal Diseases: Potential Therapeutic Applications." *Expert Opinion on Investigational Drugs* 12, no. 1 (January 2003), 39–49. www.ncbi.nlm.nih.gov/pubmed/12517253.

Dreher, M. C., K. Nugent, and R. Hudgins. "Prenatal Marijuana Exposure and Neonatal Outcomes in Jamaica: An Ethnographic Study." *Pediatrics* 93, no. 2 (February 1994): 254–60. www.ncbi.nlm.nih.gov/pubmed/8121737.

Dwyer, Devin. "Marijuana Not High Obama Priority." *ABC News*. December 14, 2012. abcnews.go.com/Politics/OTUS/president-obama-marijuana-users-high-priority-drug-war/story?id=17946783.

El-Remessy, A. B., M. Al-Shabrawey, Y. Khalifa, N. T. Tsai, R. B. Caldwell, and G. I. Liou. "Neuroprotective and Blood-Retinal Barrier Preserving Effects of Cannabidiol in Experimental Diabetes." *American Journal of Pathology* 168, no. 1 (January 2006), 235–44. www.ncbi.nlm.nih.gov/pubmed/16400026.

Elders, Joycelyn. "Myths About Medical Marijuana." *Providence Journal*. March 26, 2004.

Elzinga, S., J. Fischedick, R. Podkolinski, and J. C. Raber. "Cannabinoids and Terpenes As Chemotaxonomic Markers in Cannabis." *Natural Products Chemistry & Research* 3 (2015): 181. doi:10.4172/2329-6836.1000181.

England, T. J., W. H. Hind, N. A. Rasid, and S. E. O'Sullivan. "Cannabinoids in Experimental Stroke: A Systematic Review and Meta-Analysis." *Journal of Cerebral Blood Flow & Metabolism* 35, no. 3 (March 2015): 348–58. doi:10.1038/jcbfm.2014.218.

Eubanks, Lisa M., Claude J. Rogers, Albert E. Beuscher, George F. Koob, Arthur J. Olson, Tobin J. Dickerson, and Kim D. Janda. "A Molecular Link Between the Active Component of Marijuana and Alzheimer's Disease Pathology." *Molecular Pharmaceutics* 3, no. 6 (2006): 773–77. doi:10.1021/mp060066m.

Fishbein, M., S. Gov, F. Assaf, M. Gafni, O. Keren, and Y. Sarne. "Long-Term Behavioral and Biochemical Effects of an Ultra-Low Dose of Δ9-Tetrahydrocannabinol (THC): Neuroprotection and ERK Signaling." *Experimental Brain Research* 221, no. 4 (September 2012): 437–48. doi:10.1007/s00221-012-3186-5.

Fiz, Jimena, Marta Durán, Dolors Capellà, Jordi Carbonell, and Magí Farré. "Cannabis Use in Patients with Fibromyalgia: Effect on Symptoms Relief and Health-Related Quality of Life." *PLoS One* 6, no. 4 (April 2011), e18440. doi:10.1371/journal.pone.0018440.

Fogarty, A., P. Rawstorne, G. Prestage, J. Crawford, J. Grierson, and S. Kippax. "Marijuana As Therapy for People Living with HIV/AIDS: Social and Health Aspects." *AIDS Care* 19, no. 2 (February 2007): 295–301. www.ncbi.nlm.nih.gov/pubmed/17364413.

Fox News. "Fox News Poll: 85 Percent of Voters Favor Medical Marijuana." May 1, 2013. www.foxnews.com/politics/interactive/2013/05/01/fox-news-poll-85-percent-voters-favor-medical-marijuana/.

Fronczak, C. M., E. D. Kim, and A. B. Barqawi. "The Insults of Illicit Drug Use on Male Fertility." *Journal of Andrology* 33, no. 4 (July–August 2012): 515–28. doi:10.2164/jandrol.110.011874.

Gallily, R., Z. Yekhtin, and L. Hanuš. "Overcoming the Bell-Shaped Dose-Response of Cannabidiol by Using Cannabis Extract Enriched in Cannabidiol." *Pharmacology &*

Pharmacy 6 (2015): 75–85. doi:10.4236/pp.2015.62010.

Gorelick, David A., Kenneth H. Levin, Marc L. Copersino, Stephen J. Heishman, Fang Liu, Douglas L. Boggs, and Deanna L. Kelly. "Diagnostic Criteria for Cannabis Withdrawal Syndrome," *Drug and Alcohol Dependence* 123, no. 1–3 (June 2012): 141–47. doi:10.1016/j.drugalcdep.2011.11.007.

Grant, Igor, J. Hampton Atkinson, Ben Gouaux, and Barth Wilsey. "Medical Marijuana: Clearing Away the Smoke." *Open Neurology Journal* 6 (May 2012): 18–25. doi:10.2174/1874205X01206010018.

Greene, M. C., and J. F. Kelly. "The Prevalence of Cannabis Withdrawal and Its Influence on Adolescents' Treatment Response and Outcomes: A 12-Month Prospective Investigation." *Journal of Addiction Medicine* 8, no. 5 (September–October 2014): 359–67. doi:10.1097/ADM.0000000000000064.

Grotenhermen, F. "Pharmacokinetics and Pharmacodynamics of Cannabinoids." *Clinical Pharmacokinetics* 42, no. 4 (2003): 327–60. www.ncbi.nlm.nih.gov/pubmed/12648025.

Gupta, Sanjay. "Why I Changed My Mind on Weed." *CNN*. August 8, 2013. www.cnn.com/2013/08/08/health/gupta-changed-mind-marijuana/.

Hall, Wayne. *A Comparative Appraisal of the Health and Psychological Consequences of Alcohol, Cannabis, Nicotine, and Opiate Use.* University of New South Wales: National Drug and Alcohol Research Centre, 1995.

Hamelink, C., A. Hampson, D. A. Wink, L. E. Eiden, and R. L. Eskay. "Comparison of Cannabidiol, Antioxidants, and Diuretics in Reversing Binge Ethanol-Induced Neurotoxicity." *Journal of Pharmacology and Experimental Therapeutics* 314, no. 2 (August 2005): 780–88. www.ncbi.nlm.nih.gov/pubmed/15878999.

Huestis, Marilyn A. "Human Cannabinoid Pharmacokinetics." *Chemistry & Biodiversity* 4, no. 8 (August 2007): 1770–804. doi:10.1002/cbdv.200790152.

Jackson, S. J., L. T. Diemel, G. Pryce, and D. Baker. "Cannabinoids and Neuroprotection in CNS Inflammatory Disease." *Journal of the Neurological Sciences* 233, no. 1–2 (June 2005): 21–25. www.ncbi.nlm.nih.gov/pubmed/15894331.

Jiang, Wen, Yun Zhang, Lan Xiao, Jamie Van Cleemput, Shao-Ping Ji, Guang Bai, and Xia Zhang. "Cannabinoids Promote Embryonic and Adult Hippocampus Neurogenesis and Produce Anxiolytic and Antidepressant-like Effects." *The Journal of Clinical Investigation* 115, no. 11 (2005): 3104–16. doi:10.1172/JCI25509.

Jones, Jeffrey M. "In U.S., 58% Back Legal Marijuana Use." *Gallup*. October 21, 2015. www.gallup.com/poll/186260/back-legal-marijuana.aspx.

Karch, Steven. "Cannabis and Cardiotoxicity." *Forensic Science, Medicine, and Pathology* 2, (2006): 13–18. doi:10.1385/FSMP:2:1:13.

Karniol, I. G., I. Shirakawa, N. Kasinski, A. Pfeferman, and E. A. Carlini. "Cannabidiol Interferes with the Effects of Delta

9-Tetrahydrocannabinol in Man." *European Journal of Pharmacology* 28, no. 1 (September 1974):172–77. www.ncbi.nlm.nih.gov/pubmed/4609777.

Kassirer, Jerome P. "Federal Foolishness and Marijuana." *New England Journal of Medicine* 336, no. 5 (January 1997): 366–67. doi:10.1056/NEJM199701303360509.

Lehmann, A., L. A. Blackshaw, L. Brändén, A. Carlsson, J. Jensen, E. Nygren, and S. D. Smid. "Cannabinoid Receptor Agonism Inhibits Transient Lower Esophageal Sphincter Relaxations and Reflux in Dogs." *Gastroenterology* 123, no. 4 (October 2002), 1129–34. www.ncbi.nlm.nih.gov/pubmed/12360475.

Lotan, I., T. A. Treves, Y. Roditi, and R. Djaldetti. "Cannabis (Medical Marijuana) Treatment for Motor and Non-Motor Symptoms of Parkinson Disease: An Open-Label Observational Study." *Clinical Neuropharmacology* 37, no. 2 (March–April 2014): 41–44. doi:10.1097/WNF.0000000000000016.

Mack, Alison and Janet Joy. *Marijuana As Medicine? The Science Beyond the Controversy*. Washington DC: National Academy Press, 2001.

Martin, B. R. "Chemistry and Pharmacology of Cannabis." In: H. Kalant, W. A. Corrigall, W. Hall, R. G. Smart, eds. *The Health Effects of Cannabis*. Toronto: CAMH, 1999.

Massa, F., M. Storr, and B. Lutz. "The Endocannabinoid System in the Physiology and Pathophysiology of the Gastrointestinal Tract." *Journal of Molecular Medicine* 12, no. 1 (2005): 944–54. www.ncbi.nlm.nih.gov/pubmed/16133420.

Molina, P. E., P. Winsauer, P. Zhang, E. Walker, L. Birke, A. Amedee, C. V. Stouwe, et al. "Cannabinoid Administration Attenuates the Progression of Simian Immunodeficiency Virus." *AIDS Research and Human Retroviruses* 27, no. 6 (June 2011): 585–92. doi:10.1089/AID.2010.0218.

Müller-Vahl, Kirsten R. "Treatment of Tourette's Syndrome with Delta-9-Tetrahydrocannabinol (THC): A Randomized Crossover Trial." *Pharmacopsychiatry* 35 (2002): 57–61. doi:10.3233/BEN-120276.

National Institute on Drug Abuse. "In Nationwide Survey, More Students Use Marijuana, Fewer Use Other Drugs." April 22, 2014. www.drugabuse.gov/news-events/nida-notes/2014/04/in-nationwide-survey-more-students-use-marijuana-fewer-use-other-drugs.

National Pain Report. "Marijuana Rated Most Effective for Treating Fibromyalgia." April 21, 2014. nationalpainreport.com/marijuana-rated-most-effective-for-treating-fibromyalgia-8823638.html.

Needham, Joseph. *Science and Civilisation in China: Volume 5, Chemistry and Chemical Technology, Part 2, Spagyrical Discovery and Invention: Magisteries of Gold and Immortality*. Cambridge: Cambridge University Press, 1974.

Neff, G. W., C. B. O'Brien, K. R. Reddy, N. V. Bergasa, A. Regev, E. Molina, R. Amaro, et al. "Preliminary Observation with Dronabinol in Patients with Intractable Pruritus Secondary to Cholestatic Liver Disease." *American Journal of Gastroenterology* 97, no. 8 (August

2002): 2117–19. www.ncbi.nlm.nih.gov/pubmed/12190187.

Ngueta, G., R. E. Bélanger, E. A. Laouan, and M. Lucas. "Cannabis Use in Relation to Obesity and Insulin Resistance in the Inuit Population." *Obesity* 23, no. 2 (February 2015): 290–95. doi:10.1002/oby.20973.

Pacher, Pál, Sándor Bátkai, and George Kunos. "Blood Pressure Regulation by Endocannabinoids and Their Receptors." *Neuropharmacology* 48, no. 8 (June 2005): 1130–38. doi:10.1016/j.neuropharm.2004.12.005.

Pacher, Pál, Sándor Bátkai, and George Kunos. "The Endocannabinoid System as an Emerging Target of Pharmacotherapy." *Pharmacological Reviews* 58, no. 3 (September 2006): 389–462. www.ncbi.nlm.nih.gov/pubmed/16968947.

Passie, T., H. M. Emrich, M. Karst, S. D. Brandt, and J. H. Halpern. "Mitigation of Post-Traumatic Stress Symptoms by Cannabis Resin: A Review of the Clinical and Neurobiological Evidence." *Drug Testing and Analysis* 4, no. 7–8 (July–August 2012): 649–59. doi:10.1002/dta.1377.

PBS Frontline. "Dangerous Prescription." November 13, 2003. www.pbs.org/wgbh/pages/frontline/shows/prescription/etc/synopsis.html.

Pertwee, R. G. "Cannabinoids and the Gastrointestinal Tract." *Gut* 48, no. 6 (June 2001), 859–67. www.ncbi.nlm.nih.gov/pubmed/11358910.

Pew Research Center. "Majority Now Supports Legalizing Marijuana." April 4, 2013. www.people-press.org/2013/04/04/majority-now-supports-legalizing-marijuana/.

Piomelli, D., and E. B. Russo. "The *Cannabis sativa* versus *Cannabis indica* Debate: An Interview with Ethan Russo, MD." *Cannabis and Cannabinoid Research* 1, no. 1 (January 2016): 44–46. doi:10.1089/can.2015.29003.ebr.

Pletcher, Mark J., Eric Vittinghoff, Ravi Kalhan, Joshua Richman, Monika Safford, Stephen Sidney, Feng Lin, and Stefan Kertesz. "Association between Marijuana Exposure and Pulmonary Function over 20 Years." *Journal of American Medical Association* 307, no. 2 (January 2012):173–81. doi:10.1001/jama.2011.1961.

Powell, David, Rosalie Liccardo Pacula, and Mireille Jacobson. "Do Medical Marijuana Laws Reduce Addictions and Deaths Related to Pain Killers?" NBER Working Paper No. 21345 (July 2015). www.nber.org/papers/w21345.

Pryce, Gareth, Zubair Ahmed, Deborah J. R. Hankey, Samuel J. Jackson, J. Ludovic Croxford, Jennifer M. Pocock, Catherine Ledent, et al. "Cannabinoids Inhibit Neurodegeneration in Models of Multiple Sclerosis." *Brain* 126 (July 2003): 2191–202. doi:http://dx.doi.org/10.1093/brain/awg224.

Purohit, V., R. Rapaka, and D. Shurtleff. "Role of Cannabinoids in the Development of Fatty Liver (Steatosis)." *AAPS Journal* 12, no. 2 (June 2010): 233–37. doi:10.1208/s12248-010-9178-0.

Radjakrishnan, R., S. T. Wilkinson, and D. C. D'Souza. "Gone to Pot—A Review of the Association between Cannabis and Psychosis." *Frontiers in Psychiatry* 5 (May 2014): 54. doi:10.3389/fpsyt.2014.00054.

Richter, A. and W. Löscher. "Effects of Pharmacological Manipulations of Cannabinoid Receptors on Severe Dystonia in a Genetic Model of Paroxysmal Dyskinesia." *European Journal of Pharmacology* 454, no. 2–3 (November 2002): 145–51, www.ncbi.nlm.nih.gov/pubmed/12421641.

Romero, Dennis. "Marijuana Strains Like OG Kush Are Meaningless, Experts Say." *LA Weekly*. December 3, 2013. www.laweekly.com/news/marijuana-strains-like-og-kush-are-meaningless-expert-says-4173909.

Ryan-Ibarra, S., M. Induni, and D. Ewing. "Prevalence of Medical Marijuana Use in California, 2012." *Drug and Alcohol Review* 34, no. 2 (March 2015): 141–46. doi:10.1111/dar.12207.

Sagredo, O., M. R. Pazos, V. Satta, J. A. Ramos, R. G. Pertwee, and J. Fernández-Ruiz. "Neuroprotective Effects of Phytocannabinoid-Based Medicines in Experimental Models of Huntington's Disease." *Journal of Neuroscience Research* 89, no. 9 (September 2011): 1509–18. doi:10.1002/jnr.22682.

Sarafaraz, Sami, Vaqar M. Adhami, Deeba N. Syed, Farrukh Afaq, and Hasan Mukhtar. "Cannabinoids for Cancer Treatment: Progress and Promise." *Cancer Research* 68 (January 2008): 339–42. doi:10.1158/0008-5472.CAN-07-2785.

Sido, J. M., P. S. Nagarkatti, and M. Nagarkatti. "Δ9-Tetrahydrocannabinol Attenuates Allogeneic Host-Versus-Graft Response and Delays Skin Graft Rejection Through Activation of Cannabinoid Receptor 1 and Induction of Myeloid-Derived Suppressor Cells." *Journal of Leukocyte Biology* 98, no. 3 (September 2015): 435–47. doi:10.1189/jlb.3A0115-030RR.

Sirven, J. I. "Marijuana for Epilepsy: Winds of Change." *Epilepsy & Behavior* 29, no. 3 (December 2013): 435–36. doi:10.1016/j.yebeh.2013.09.004.

Smith, S. C., and M. S. Wagner. "Clinical Endocannabinoid Deficiency (CECD) Revisited: Can This Concept Explain the Therapeutic Benefits of Cannabis in Migraine, Fibromyalgia, Irritable Bowel Syndrome and Other Treatment-Resistant Conditions?" *Neuro Endocrinology Letters* 35, no. 3 (2014): 198–201. www.ncbi.nlm.nih.gov/pubmed/24977967.

Szepietowski, J. C., T. Szepietowski, and A. Reich. "Efficacy and Tolerance of the Cream Containing Structured Physiological Lipid Endocannabinoids in the Treatment of Uremic Pruritus: A Preliminary Study." *Acta Dermatovenerologic Croatica* 13, no. 2 (2005): 97–103. www.ncbi.nlm.nih.gov/pubmed/16324422.

United States Drug Enforcement Agency. "Drug Scheduling." Accessed December 27, 2015. www.dea.gov/druginfo/ds.shtml.

University of Pittsburgh Medical Center. "Marijuana-Derived Drug Suppresses Bladder Pain in Animal Models." May 21, 2006.

Vanity Fair, Volume 5, January 4, 1862.

Wade, D. T., P. Robson, H. House, P. Makela, and J. Aram. "A Preliminary Controlled Study to Determine Whether Whole-Plant Cannabis Extracts Can Improve Intractable Neurogenic Symptoms." *Clinical Rehabilitation* 17, no. 1 (February 2003): 21–29. www.ncbi.nlm.nih.gov/pubmed/12617376.

Waissengrin, B., D. Urban, Y. Leshem, M. Garty, and I. Wolf. "Patterns of Use of Medical Cannabis Among Israeli Cancer Patients: A Single Institution Experience." *Journal of Pain and Symptom Management* 49, no. 2 (February 2015): 223–30. doi:10.1016 /j.jpainsymman.2014.05.018.

Wallace, M. S., T. D. Marcotte, A. Umlauf, B. Gouaux, and J. H. Atkinson. "Efficacy of Inhaled Cannabis on Painful Diabetic Neuropathy." *The Journal of Pain* 16, no. 7 (July 2015), 616–27. doi:10.1016 /j.jpain.2015.03.008.

Wargent, E. T., M. S. Zaibi, C. Silvestri, D. C. Hislop, C. J. Stocker, C. G. Stott, G. W. Guy, et al. "The Cannabinoid Δ9-Tetrahydrocannabivarin (THCV) Ameliorates Insulin Sensitivity in Two Mouse Models of Obesity." *Nutrition & Diabetes* 3 (May 2013): e68. doi:10.1038 /nutd.2013.9.

WebMD. "Legalize Medical Marijuana, Doctors Say in Survey." April 2, 2014. www.webmd.com/news/breaking-news /marijuana-on-main-street/20140225 /webmd-marijuana-survey-web.

Weiss, L., M. Zeira, S. Reich, M. Har-Noy, R. Mechoulam, S. Slavin, and R. Gallily. "Cannabidiol Lowers Incidence of Diabetes in Non-Obese Diabetic Mice." *Autoimmunity* 39, no. 2 (March 2006): 143–51. www.ncbi .nlm.nih.gov/pubmed/16698671.

Winterborne, Jeffrey. *Medical Marijuana Cannabis Cultivation: Trees of Life at the University of London.* Guildford, UK: Pukka Press, 2008.

Wright, K., N. Rooney, M. Feeney, J. Tate, D. Robertson, M. Welham, and S. Ward. "Differential Expression of Cannabinoid Receptors in the Human Colon: Cannabinoids Promote Epithelial Wound Healing." *Gastroenterology* 129, no. 2 (August 2005): 437–53. www.ncbi.nlm.nih.gov/pubmed/16083701.

Young, Francis L. "In the Matter of Marijuana Rescheduling Petition; Docket No. 86-22." September 6, 1988. www.ccguide.org /young88.php.

SYMPTOMS & AILMENTS INDEX

Throughout this book, we reference a variety of symptoms or ailments that might be easier to manage with cannabis. We've gathered these references here so you that if you're suffering from a particular ailment or symptom, you can look up whatever information we've presented about it. In addition, we've noted pages that reference the symptom in relation to delivery methods, cannabis compounds or strains, and recipes.

mood disorders and
  cannabinoids, 40
multiple sclerosis (MS), 166
  cannabinoids, 40
  hybrid strains, 92, 95, 97–98
  indica strains, 73
  research, 32
muscle pain and essential oil
  blends, 125
muscle relaxers and myrcene, 20
muscle spasms
  cannabinoids, 40, 41
  indica strains, 73
muscle tension
  indica strains, 78

N

nausea
  cannabinoids, 40
  hybrid strains, 92–95, 97–100
  indica strains, 72–75, 77–78
  reducing, 28
  research, 31–32
  sativa strains, 83–89
neurodegenerative diseases
  and cannabinoids, 41
neuropathic pain
  cannabinoids, 40
  relieving, 28
  research, 32
neuropathy
  hybrid strains, 98

O

osteoporosis research, 36

P

pain, 132, 166
  cannabinoids, 40, 41
  dogs, 18
  hybrid strains, 92–99
  indica strains, 72, 76, 79
  sativa strains, 82–89
painkillers and myrcene, 20
pain relief
  essential oil blends, 125
  indica strains, 72–79
  terpenes, 42

Parkinson's disease
  cannabinoids, 40
  hybrid strains, 95
  indica strains, 74
  research, 33
PMS
  hybrid strains, 95, 97, 100
  indica strains, 75, 77
posttraumatic stress
  disease (PTSD)
  cannabidiol (CBD), 20
  hybrid strains, 92, 96–98, 100
  indica strains, 72, 75, 77, 79
  relaxing, 28
  research, 34–35
  sativa strains, 82–85, 88
pregnancy and cannabis, 37, 45
pruritus (itching)
  cannabinoids, 40
  research, 35

R

relaxation and essential oil
  blends, 125
rheumatism and ancient use
  of cannabis, 17
rheumatoid arthritis research, 32

S

schizophrenia and
  cannabinoids, 40
sedatives and myrcene, 20
seizure disorder, 11, 59
  cannabinoids, 40
  hybrid strains, 94, 96–97
  sativa strains, 89
sleep apnea
  cannabinoids, 40
  indica strains, 76
  research, 36
sleep disorders
  hybrid strains, 93, 95–96,
  98, 100
  indica strains, 72–75, 77
  sativa strains, 88
soothing relief and essential
  oil blends, 125

spasticity
  hybrid strains, 94, 97–98
  sativa strains, 83
spinal cord injury
  chronic nerve pain, 32
  hybrid strains, 95–96, 99
stress
  hybrid strains, 92–100
  indica strains, 72–79
  sativa strains, 82–89
stroke research, 33

T

teenagers' changes in brain, 45
Tourette syndrome
  cannabinoids, 40
  hybrid strains, 96
  research, 35
transplants, rejecting candidates
  using cannabis, 44
tumors and cannabigerol
  (CBG), 20

U

ulcers and terpenes, 42
urinary incontinence research, 34

V

viral throat infections and
  smoking marijuana, 49

INDEX

ACKNOWLEDGMENTS

WE ARE DEEPLY GRATEFUL for all the patients, doctors, and industry folks who gave us their time, stories, and support. A very special thanks to those who gave us permission to include their testimonies in this book. We hope these stories will inspire others to ask questions and seek new treatments to improve their health and the health of their loved ones.

We would also like to thank Meg, Clara, Carol, Amanda, and the team at Callisto Media for their constant support, patience, and encouragement in the creation of this book. Without these folks, this book would not have happened. Thanks go out to Ricardo, Aleta, Megan, Selena, Tyler, Alex, Nicole, and the folks at Verdabase for their industry insights and knowledge—you guys rock!

We are grateful to have family and dear friends who have helped and supported our efforts along the way. A special thank you to Bruce and Nick, the men in our lives who have supported our work in the cannabis industry from the beginning.

PHOTO CREDITS

ABOUT THE AUTHORS

LAURIE AND MARY WOLF are a mother and daughter-in-law team. Together, they run the award-winning cannabis company, Laurie & MaryJane, which produces a popular line of medical marijuana edibles. In addition to producing high-quality edibles for medical marijuana dispensaries, they provide recipes and guidance for at-home edible creations. When producing edibles and recipes, their goal is to provide high-quality products that help patients medicate safely and effectively.

LAURIE, a classically trained chef and graduate of the Culinary Institute of America, has been a food stylist, food editor, recipe developer, and cookbook author for over 30 years. She is a regular contributor and edible recipe developer for *The Cannabist*, *High Times*, *Oregon Leaf*, and *Cannabis Now* and a leader in the art of marijuana edibles. Laurie's passion for cannabis as a part of therapeutic treatment stems from her exposure to its use in her father's end-of-life care, as well as its use in the successful management of her seizure disorder. Laurie also works with hospice groups, veterans with PTSD, and other patients who seek safe, compassionate care for their health problems.

MARY left a marketing and research career at a New York investment firm specializing in innovative medical treatments and moved to Portland where she partnered with Laurie to build Laurie & MaryJane. Through her experience in providing treatment for medical marijuana patients with a range of ailments, as well as her expertise from years of accumulated research, Mary has become an advocate for medical marijuana and cannabis legalization. In addition to running a thriving company together, Mary and Laurie have written several books on cooking with cannabis. Learn more about Laurie and Mary at laurieandmaryjane.com.